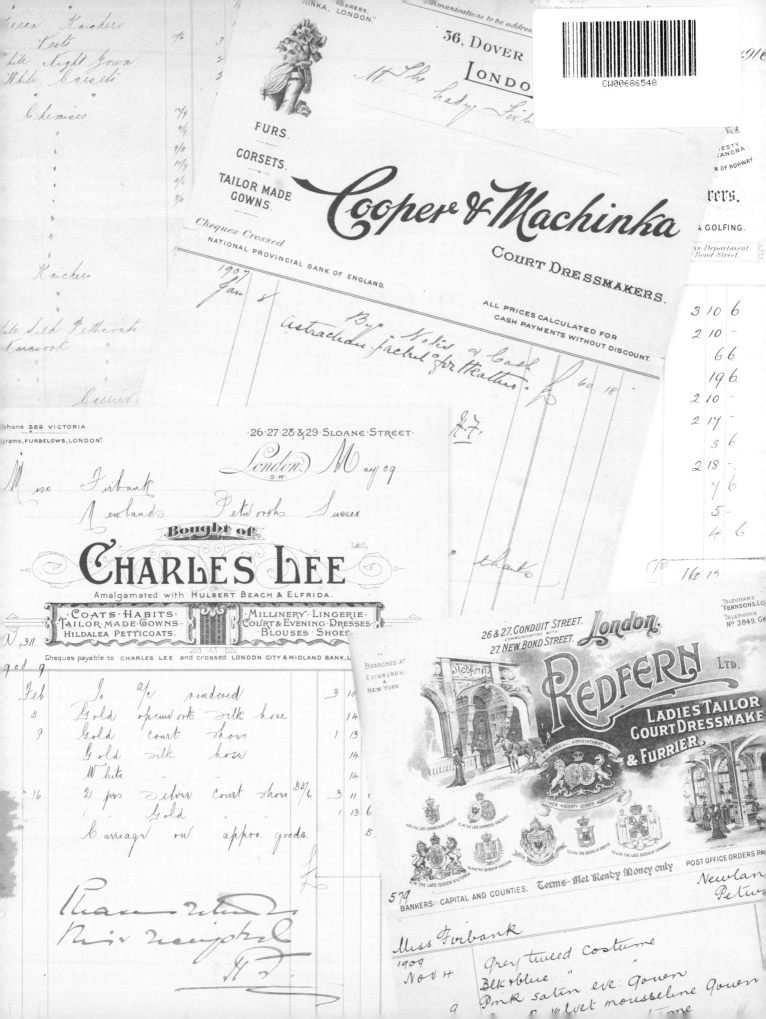

Green Knickers
Vests   1/6   3
Silk Night Gown   3
White Corsets   3

Chemises   17/9

"   11/9
"   9/10
"   10/4
"   6/6
"   9/6

Knickers

Blue Silk Petticoat
Nainsook "

Carried

FURS.
CORSETS.
TAILOR MADE
GOWNS.

Cheques Crossed
NATIONAL PROVINCIAL BANK OF ENGLAND.

Cooper & Machinka
COURT DRESSMAKERS.

ALL PRICES CALCULATED FOR
CASH PAYMENTS WITHOUT DISCOUNT.

1907
Jan 8

By Notes & Cash
Astrachan Jacket for Weather £ 60 18 -

3 10 6
2 10 -
6 6
19 6
2 10 -
2 17 -
3 6
2 18 -
7 6
5 -
4 6

16 15

Phone 389 VICTORIA
Grams, FURBELOWS, LONDON."

26·27·28·& 29·SLOANE·STREET·
London. May 09
S.W.

Miss Firbank
Newlands Petworth Sussex

Bought of
CHARLES LEE
Ltd.
Amalgamated with HULBERT BEACH & ELFRIDA.

COATS·HABITS·   MILLINERY·LINGERIE·
TAILOR·MADE·GOWNS·   COURT & EVENING·DRESSES·
HILDALEA PETTICOATS.   BLOUSES·SHOES·

N 311.

Cheques payable to CHARLES LEE and crossed LONDON CITY & MIDLAND BANK, L

1908 9

Feb   To   a/c   rendered   3 10
5   Gold   open work silk hose   14
8   Gold   court shoes   1 13
  Gold   silk hose   14
  White   14
16   2 prs silver court shoes   35/6   3 11
  1 " Gold "   1 13 6
  Carriage on appro. goods.   5

BRANCHES AT
EDINBURGH
&
NEW YORK.

26 & 27. CONDUIT STREET.
COMMUNICATING WITH
27. NEW BOND STREET.

London.

TELEGRAMS
"FERNSONS, LO
TELEPHONE
No 3849. G

REDFERN
LTD.
LADIES TAILOR
COURT DRESSMAKER
& FURRIER.

BY SPECIAL APPOINTMENT TO
HER MAJESTY QUEEN ALEXANDRA

H.R.H. THE LATE GRAND DUKE HESSE   H.I.M. THE LATE EMPRESS FREDERIC

TO H.M. THE QUEEN OF PORTUGAL   TO H.M. THE QUEEN OF GREECE   TO H.M. THE LATE QUEEN OF DENMARK

H.M. THE LATE QUEEN VICTORIA

579
BANKERS: CAPITAL AND COUNTIES.   Terms—Net Ready Money only.   POST OFFICE ORDERS PA

Newlan
Petw

Miss Firbank
1909   Grey tweed Costume
Nov 4   Blk & blue "
  Pink satin eve. gown
9   velvet mousseline gown

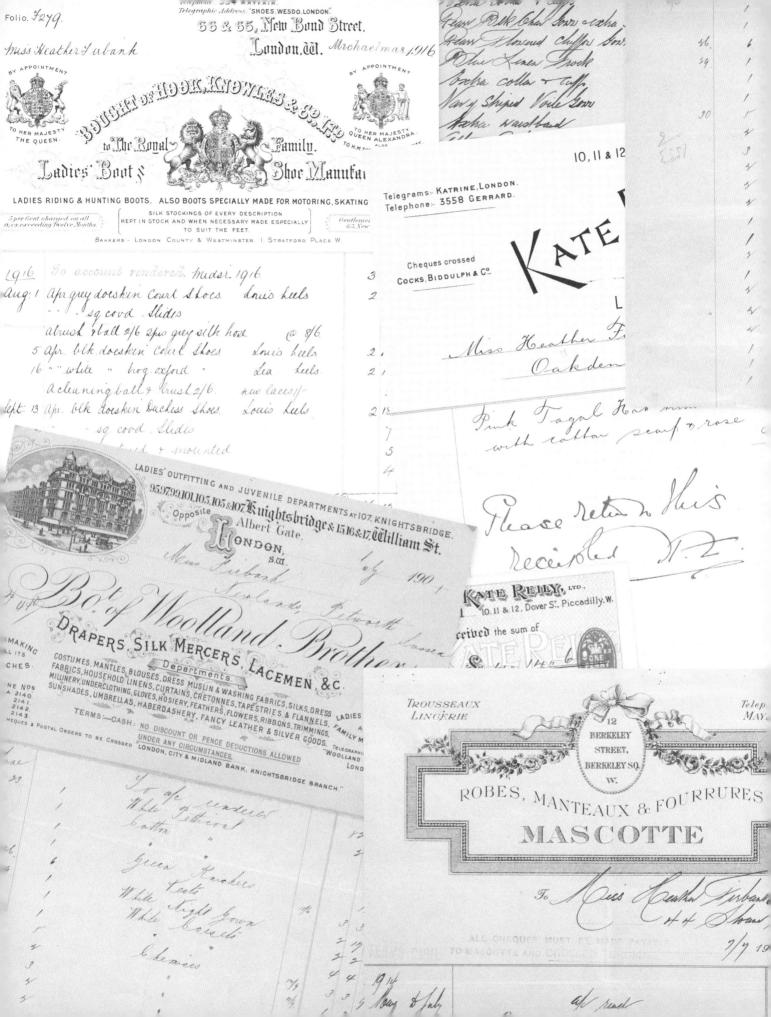

Folio. 7279.

Telegraphic Address "SHOES, WESDO, LONDON."

66 & 65, New Bond Street.
London, W. Michaelmas, 1916

Miss Heather Firbank

BOUGHT OF HOOK, KNOWLES & CO. LTD
to The Royal Family.
Ladies' Boot & Shoe Manufac

BY APPOINTMENT TO HER MAJESTY THE QUEEN

BY APPOINTMENT TO HER MAJESTY QUEEN ALEXANDRA. ALSO TO H.M.T...

LADIES RIDING & HUNTING BOOTS. ALSO BOOTS SPECIALLY MADE FOR MOTORING, SKATING

5 per Cent charged on all a/cs exceeding Twelve Months.

SILK STOCKINGS OF EVERY DESCRIPTION
KEPT IN STOCK AND WHEN NECESSARY MADE ESPECIALLY
TO SUIT THE FEET.

Gentlemen 64 New

BANKERS - LONDON COUNTY & WESTMINSTER. I, STRATFORD PLACE W.

1916 To account rendered Midsr. 1916

Aug. 1 Apr grey doeskin court shoes. Louis heels
" ... sq covd Slides
a brush & ball 2/6 2 prs grey silk hose @ 8/6
5 Apr. blk. doeskin court shoes. Louis heels
16 " white " hog. oxford . Lea heels
a cleaning ball & brush 2/6 new laces/f
Sept. 13 Apr. blk. doeskin Duchess shoes. Louis heels
" sq covd. Slides
tried & mounted

Telegrams - KATRINE, LONDON.
Telephone - 3558 GERRARD.

10, 11 & 12

Cheques crossed
Cocks, Biddulph & Co.

KATE R

L

Miss Heather F

Oakden

Pink Tagal Hat...
with cotton scarf & rose

Please return this
Receipted H.F.

KATE REILLY, LTD.,
10, 11 & 12, Dover St., Piccadilly. W.
received the sum of

LADIES' OUTFITTING AND JUVENILE DEPARTMENTS AT 107, KNIGHTSBRIDGE.
95, 97, 99, 101, 103, 105 & 107 Knightsbridge & 15, 16 & 17, William St.
Opposite Albert Gate,
LONDON, S.W.

Miss Firbank

Newlands, Petworth, Sussex

Bot of Woolland Brothers
DRAPERS, SILK MERCERS, LACEMEN, &C.
Departments

COSTUMES, MANTLES, BLOUSES, DRESS MUSLIN & WASHING FABRICS, SILKS, DRESS
FABRICS, HOUSEHOLD LINENS, CURTAINS, CRETONNES, TAPESTRIES, & FLANNELS,
MILLINERY, UNDERCLOTHING, GLOVES, HOSIERY, FEATHERS, FLOWERS, RIBBONS, TRIMMINGS,
SUNSHADES, UMBRELLAS, HABERDASHERY, FANCY LEATHER & SILVER GOODS.

LADIES A...
FAMILY M...

TERMS:—CASH; NO DISCOUNT OR PENCE DEDUCTIONS ALLOWED
UNDER ANY CIRCUMSTANCES.

CHEQUES & POSTAL ORDERS TO BE CROSSED LONDON, CITY & MIDLAND BANK, KNIGHTSBRIDGE BRANCH.

Telegraphic "Woolland Lond

To a/c rendered
White Petticoat
Cotton "
Green Knickers
Vests
White Night Gown
White Corsets "
Chemises

TROUSSEAUX
LINGÈRIE

12
BERKELEY
STREET,
BERKELEY SQ.
W.

Telep
MAY

ROBES, MANTEAUX & FOURRURES
MASCOTTE

To Miss Heather Firbank
44 Sloane

ALL CHEQUES MUST BE MADE PAYABLE
TO MASCOTTE AND CROSSED LONDON

7/7 19

1914
May & July

LONDON SOCIETY FASHION
1905–1925

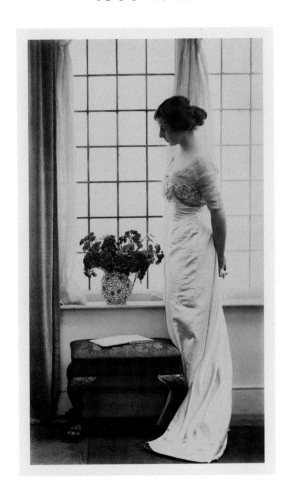

THE WARDROBE OF
HEATHER FIRBANK

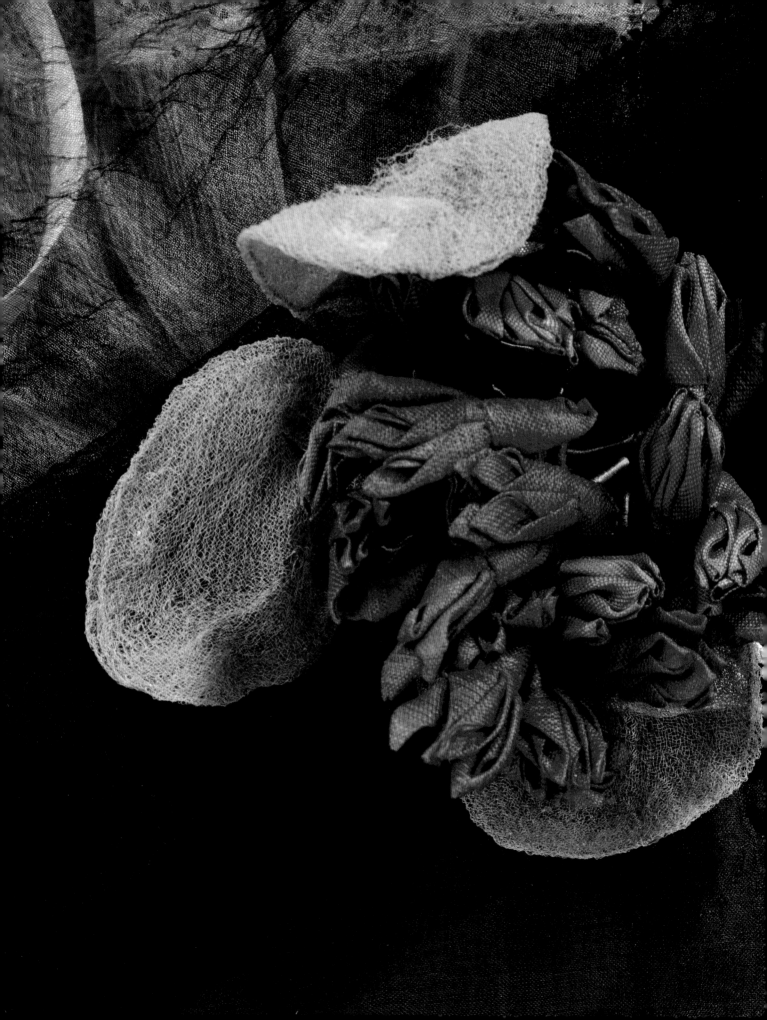

CASSIE DAVIES-STRODDER

JENNY LISTER AND

LOU TAYLOR

V&A PUBLISHING

London Society Fashion
1905 / 1925
THE WARDROBE OF HEATHER FIRBANK

First published by V&A Publishing, 2015
Victoria and Albert Museum
South Kensington
London SW7 2RL
www.vandapublishing.com

Distributed in North America by Abrams,
an imprint of ABRAMS

ISBN 978 1 85177 831 7

Library of Congress Control Number 2014951845

10 9 8 7 6 5 4 3 2 1
2018 2017 2016 2015

Designed and typeset in Fleischman by Dalrymple
Copy-editor: Lesley Levene
Indexer: Hilary Bird

Front jacket illustration: detail of plate 83.

Back jacket illustrations (clockwise from top): plates 1, 46 (detail),
75, 153, 137.

Front flap illustration: detail of plate 138.

Back flap illustrations: plate 34 (top), plate 53 (bottom).

Endpapers: A selection of bills from the Heather Firbank archive.

Page 1: Heather Firbank, photographed by Lallie Charles, London,
c.1908. V&A: Heather Firbank archive.

Pages 2–3: detail of plate 42.

V&A photography by the V&A Photographic Studio

Printed in China

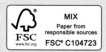

V&A Publishing

Supporting the world's leading
museum of art and design,
the Victoria and Albert
Museum, London

CONTENTS

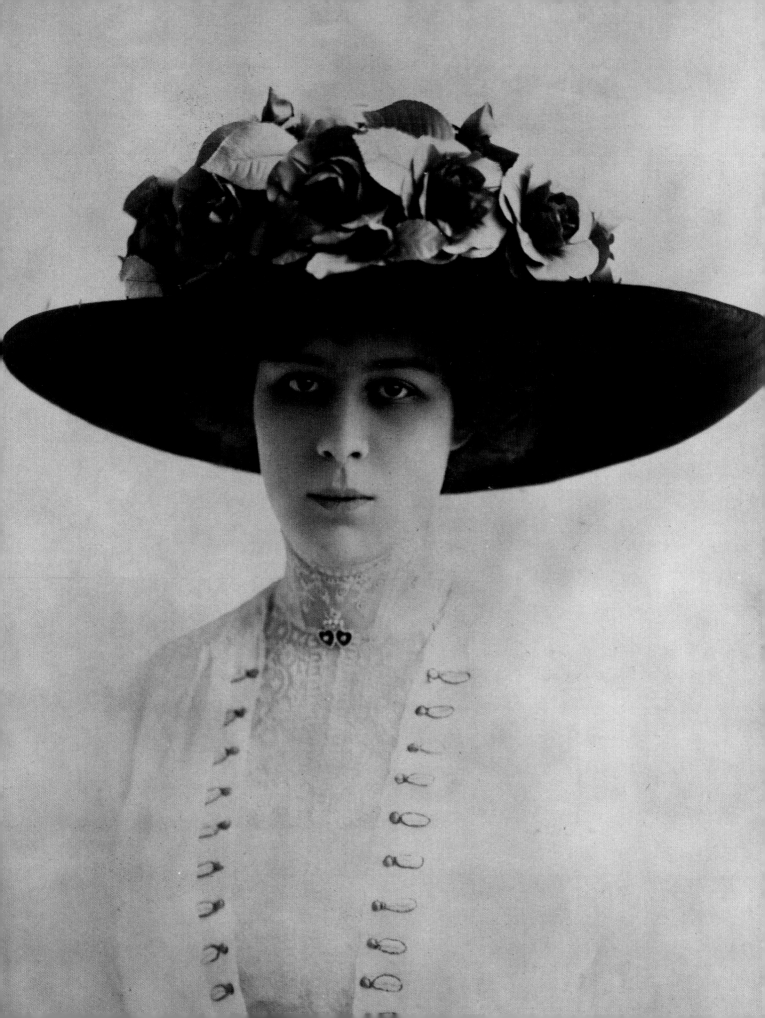

INTRODUCTION

Heather Firbank (1888–1954) was a remarkably fashionable young woman who moved in London society in the decade leading up to the First World War. In 1926, Heather packed away her extensive wardrobe of fine clothes, bought from the very best dressmakers and tailors in London. These treasures remained undiscovered for over 30 years until, after her death, over 200 items were acquired by the Victoria and Albert Museum, laying the foundations for the V&A's now world-famous fashion collection. Society circles were accessible only to those of aristocratic background or with immense wealth, and within such circles great emphasis was placed on a woman's appearance. Heather required specific garments for the wide range of activities making up the whirl of social events known as 'the season' to comply with expected codes of etiquette-correct dress and detailed rules concerning manners and behaviour.

Clothing from this period is often fragile and is as ephemeral as the passing fashions themselves, making this an exceptionally large collection of historic dress to survive from one person's wardrobe. Dating from between 1905 and the mid-1920s, it encompasses everything from fine couture evening gowns, hats and superbly tailored daywear to underwear, gloves and stockings. Significant changes in fashion – including the move from the separate bodices and skirts of 1901–7 to the increasingly slimline one-piece dresses of 1908–12; the growing importance of the tailored costume and separate blouse and skirt; and finally the loss of all boning and shape in the simpler garments of the 1920s – are all reflected in the clothes which survive. Alongside the clothes, the Museum acquired a large quantity of related bills and ephemera [2], including Heather's correspondence with the fashion houses she patronized, her cuttings from fashion magazines and newspapers, and several studio photographs of her taken in her early twenties. This material now forms the Heather Firbank archive at the V&A's Archive of Art and Design.

This collection provides a rare, remarkably complete picture of one fashionable young woman's tastes and shopping habits in the early twentieth century. It also tells us much about the clothes' wearer, Heather Firbank.

REVEALING HEATHER'S STORY

Heather Firbank has always been in the shadow of her well-known collection of clothes and her much more famous brother, avant-garde author and playwright Ronald Firbank. Here for the first time it is her story which is in focus. In 1908 Heather Firbank was launched as a young debutante, with the privileged future as a married aristocrat and society hostess that this promised. However, her life took a very different turn. The loss of the family's wealth and a scandalous love affair in her early twenties had a profound impact on her options. She never married and spent her later life moving between hotels and women's clubs.

Through all of this Heather was a keen follower of fashion. She was an avid reader of fashion features in magazines and newspapers and, being tall, slender and attractive, was the ideal model for the exquisite, expensive garments she purchased. Her taste was refined and largely restrained. She favoured pared-down garments in mauve and purple hues,

1 Heather Firbank wearing hat in plate 3, probably photographed by Lallie Charles, London, c.1908
V&A: HEATHER FIRBANK ARCHIVE

TELEPHONE Nº 2885 GERRARD. (3 LINES)
TELEGRAMS GRACEFULLY, LONDON.

London, W.   Dec 16 1909

Mrs Firbank

Newlands, Petworth

Sussex

To Reville & Rossiter LTD

15 & 16 · Hanover Square ·

Terms.- PROMPT CASH WITHOUT DISCOUNT.

35A

IT IS PARTICULARLY REQUESTED THAT ALL COMMUNICATIONS BE ADDRESSED TO THE FIRM.

1908				
Dec 21	Ivory satin evening gown	22 gns	23	2
1909				
Jany 6	Diamond headdress	3	3	3
"	Pearl "	2	2	2
July 15	White linen coat skirt	6	6	6
" 31	Yellow linen coat skirt	6	6	6
Nov 11	Pink satin evening gown	20	21	.
Dec 3	Cleaning renovating evening gown 2		2	2
			64	1
	12.09 on a/c		21	10
	Balance		42	11

Nº 5875   15 & 16. Hanover Square. W.

Received with thanks
Reville & Rossiter LTD

ONE PENNY

£ 21 - 10 - 0 on a/c

16/12/09

Per S. Clarke.

made by a select group of the very best dressmakers and tailors and purchased almost exclusively in London. Although her wardrobe forms a cohesive and recognizable whole, there are notable variations in her style. Girlish, slightly fussy garments survive from her adolescence (1905–7); more refined, pared-down, sophisticated garments from her early twenties (1908–10); and a group of alluring and refined gowns from her mid-twenties (1910–13). Less clothing and no photographs of Heather's survive from around the time of the First World War, and in what was kept almost no evening wear and very little colour feature. Although influenced by changing trends, these clothing choices were above all personal to Heather and reflect her maturing age and changing circumstances.

Through surviving letters and photographs, Heather emerges as a woman at once aware of the frivolity and superficiality of maintaining a fashionable appearance while also being seemingly unable or unwilling to resist spending vast amounts of money on fine clothing. Perhaps this preoccupation provided welcome distraction for her. Tinged with great loss and unfulfilled promises of happiness, Heather's life story is ultimately one of misfortune, and her letters show her at times to be overwhelmed by sadness, lonely and isolated. Her story does much to reveal how restricted her options were as a single woman in the period leading up to the First World War, and how vulnerable and reliant on others she was in matters of finance, acquaintances, accommodation and travel.

ONE WOMAN'S WARDROBE: A CASE STUDY
Much is revealed by focusing on one woman's life and surviving wardrobe, but much also remains obscure. Heather's surviving clothing dates from a period of great change in both society and fashion, and inevitably this case study is limited in what it can show of these changes. With no surviving diaries or reflections from Heather in memoirs, extracts from those of her contemporaries (such as Lady Lucy Duff-Gordon and Cynthia Asquith) and those who

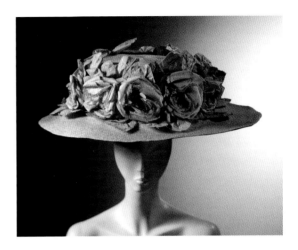

grew up in the period (such as Cecil Beaton) are needed to shed light on the context of her passion for fashionable dress and to describe the social scene in which she wore it. As there is little or no evidence of Heather taking part in the campaign for women's suffrage or women's work during the two world wars – movements so crucial to the society and politics of this period – these issues are not the focus here.

Rather than providing a broad-brush historical survey, the Heather Firbank Collection allows us to concentrate on the life and tastes of a single, wealthy, fashionable woman. This book uses Heather's clothes and papers to explore changing fashions, the experience of shopping, and the dressmakers and department stores of the period, drawing on complementary sources including Post Office directories, census returns and newspapers to reconstruct histories of once grand, now forgotten London dressmakers.

'DRESS WAS A NEW PRIORITY'
The story of the Heather Firbank Collection at the V&A is inextricably linked to the story of the Textiles and Fashion Department at the Museum. The collection was accepted in 1957 by the very first Curator of Dress, Madeleine Ginsburg, when fashion as a form of fine and decorative art was not as highly regarded in the Museum as it is today. As Ginsburg recalls,

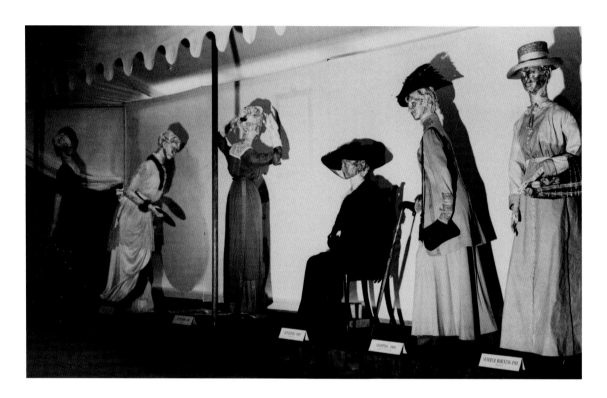

'We never had any freedom. Dress was a new priority. It had nothing in common with antiquities and intellect – it was a battle.'[1] Great credit must be given to Ginsburg for acquiring so much of the Firbank gift in this climate. Her early research into Edwardian dressmakers, including correspondence with relatives of the makers still alive in the late 1950s, provided a starting point for the investigation into the world of London court dressmakers presented here and has been invaluable in the study of twentieth-century dress at the V&A.

Madeleine Ginsburg sorted through the surviving garments with Heather's former lady's maid, Adelaide Hallett, but was not able to take everything. Once Ginsburg had selected what she wanted for the V&A's collections, the trunks of remaining clothes began a tour of UK museums. Pieces were acquired by the Gallery of English Costume in Manchester (now the Gallery of Costume), Nottingham Museum and Leicester Museum. Incredibly, what was taken in

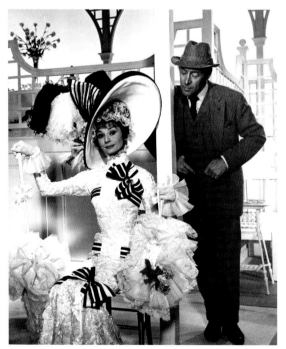

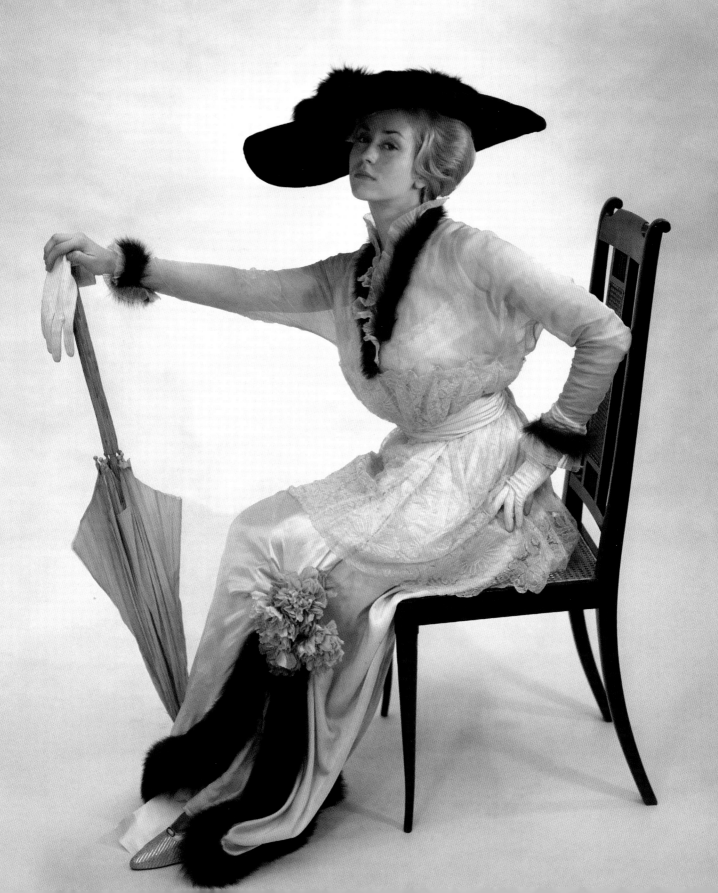

6 Actress Ann Firbank (a distant relative of the Firbank family) wearing the dress in plate 84, photographed by Cecil Beaton, 1962
NATIONAL PORTRAIT GALLERY, LONDON

by museums at this time – almost 250 items – was only half of what survived from this 20-year period of Heather's life: the remaining items from Heather's wardrobe were sold by her great-nieces in 1974 at an auction at Christie's. At this sale garments and accessories were acquired by the London Museum (now the Museum of London), Northampton Museum and again Nottingham Museum.[2] Numerous other items of dress were sold into private ownership, some to be used as props in stage and film productions.[3] Despite the richness of what was offered for sale and to museums – over 400 pieces from a period of just 20 years – these numerous surviving garments still do not represent all that Heather owned and wore at this time. Many more items of dress from the 1910s and 1920s are listed in surviving dressmakers' bills, providing a glimpse of just how large her total wardrobe would have been.

The collection at the V&A has been used extensively since its acquisition in 1957. Items from Heather's wardrobe have appeared in every single permanent display in the fashion galleries since they opened in 1962. Several pieces from the collection formed the basis of a touring exhibition entitled *Edwardian Elegance* which was loaned by the Museum's (now defunct) Circulation Department 21 times in four years to venues all across the UK. Heather's exceptional hats were shown in the exhibition *Hats: An Anthology by Stephen Jones* and photographs of her clothes have featured in numerous publications. The most focused use of the V&A collection to date, however, was the exhibition of Heather's clothing staged just after it was acquired, in 1960. Entitled *A Lady of Fashion: Heather Firbank and What She Wore between 1908 and 1921*, this was the first major display of twentieth-century fashionable dress to be held at the V&A. Although many in the Museum had to be convinced that this was a worthwhile subject, the exhibition was a huge success and its run was extended to accommodate the demand from visitors.[4] *A Lady of Fashion*, curated by Madeleine Ginsburg, drew attention to the appeal of fashionable dress for the Museum and deserves to be acknowledged alongside Cecil Beaton's *Fashion: An Anthology* in 1971 for its role in putting fashion on the map at the V&A [4].

In keeping with the Museum's original purpose as a resource for research and an inspiration for designers, items of Heather's clothing which are not on display have been studied by historians and contemporary designers alike. Most notably, influences from the collection, which was photographed by Cecil Beaton in 1960, can be seen in his costume designs for the 1964 film *My Fair Lady* [5, 6]. More recently, Susannah Buxton, costume designer for *Downton Abbey* (series 1 and 2), has cited the collection as an 'invaluable resource', and was fascinated to find parallels between Heather's story and those of characters in the television series. Despite this extensive use, during the more than 50-year history of Heather's clothes at the Museum what has remained neglected is the story of Heather's life. With the added archive of photographs, letters and account books generously shared by Heather's last surviving descendant, her great-niece Johanna Firbank, we aim to reunite the clothes with the untold story of their wearer, celebrating the central role of fashion in Heather's life.

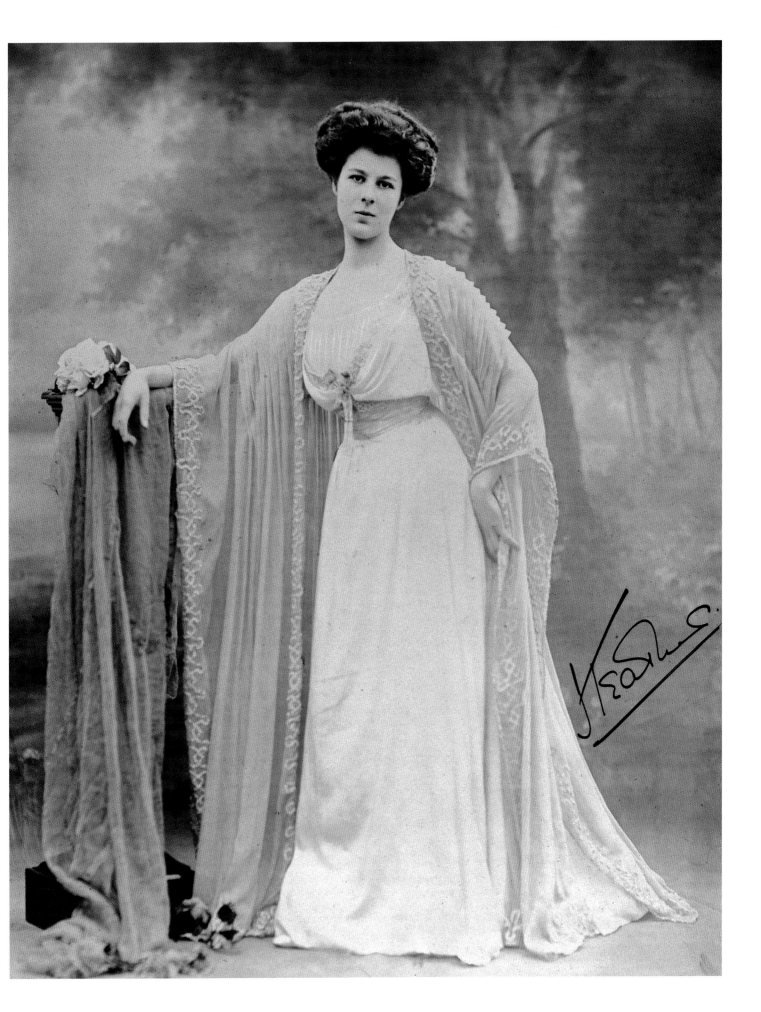

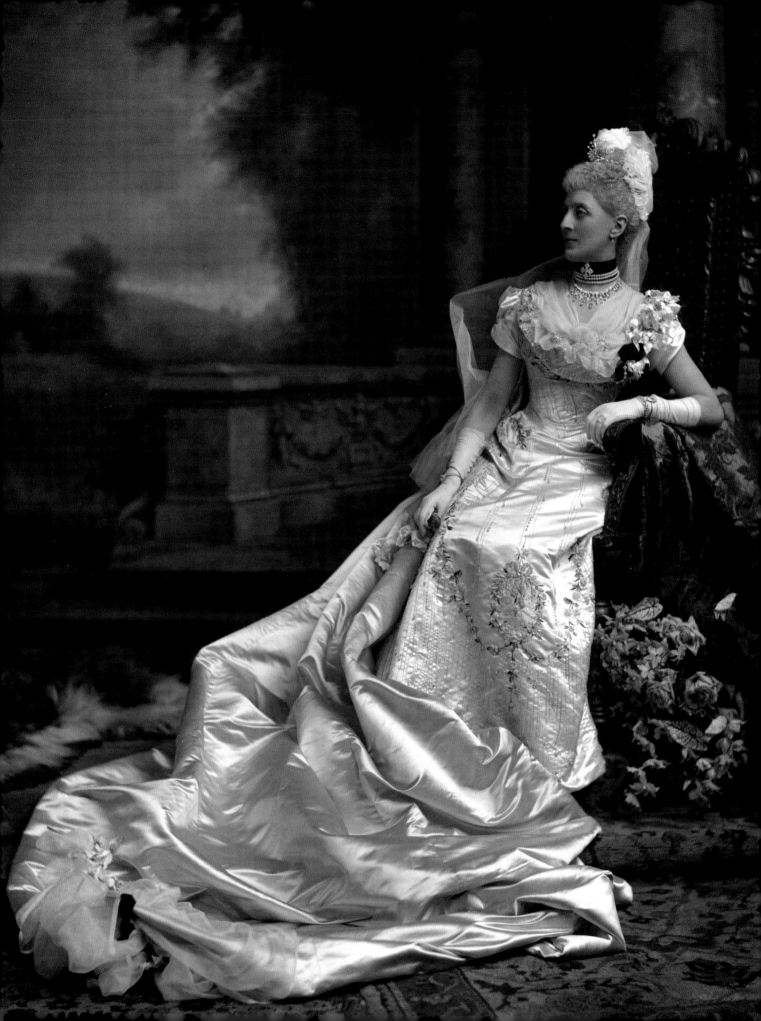

A SPLENDID CRESCENDO OF LUXURY:
CHILDHOOD AND THE FIRBANK FAMILY
1901-8

With the death of Queen Victoria on 22 January 1901, Edward VII came to the throne, bringing with him an endorsement of all things fashionable. In his long service as Prince of Wales, Edward had built a reputation as a pleasure seeker. He and his friends, known as the Marlborough House Set after his London residence, were famous for their parties, while he and his wife, Alexandra, loved clothes, were leaders of taste and spent considerable time and money on their wardrobes. The new era was highly fashion-conscious, with an increased emphasis for women on pastel colours and delicate textiles. However, though lighter in appearance, women's dresses remained built over a restrictive foundation of corsetry that reached from under the bust to the hips, forcing bodies into the forward tilt of an 'S' bend.

Heather Firbank was 13 at the coronation of Edward VII in 1902. The most fashionable period of her life was to be played out in the years that followed, up to the First World War. This was a time later vividly described by the society restaurateur and interior designer Marcel Boulestin: 'Those years, 1908–1911, seem to have a certain historical value as the prelude to a new era, like a splendid crescendo of luxury, pleasure, happiness, artistic glory, opening with the glow of the Coronation and finishing fortissimo in August 1914 when the first guns sounded the knell of civilisation.'[1]

CHILDHOOD AND THE FIRBANK FAMILY
Although often seen as a period which broke down many of the social barriers of the Victorian era, the early twentieth century remained bound by a strict hierarchy, and an individual's status was still measured by family background and wealth. Understanding the Firbanks' social standing is crucial to

placing Heather and her surviving garments in context.

Heather was a member of a wealthy upper-middle-class London family whose fortune came from her grandfather Joseph Firbank, a railway contractor from a mining family in County Durham. Having made his fortune converting canals into railways in South Wales, Joseph was able to educate his son Joseph Thomas Firbank (known as Thomas) at Cheltenham College, a respected boys' public school. Boosted by his upper-middle-class education, in 1883 Thomas Firbank married Harriette Jane Garrett, a member of the well-established and aristocratic Annesley family, who could trace their ancestry in Ireland back to Sir Francis Annesley, Baron Mountnorris and 1st Viscount Valentia (1585–1660). It was thanks to her mother's and grandmother's Anglo-Irish aristocratic connections that Heather was guaranteed entrée into court circles [8].

Thomas and Harriette Firbank spent the first years of their married life living in fashionable Clarges Street in Mayfair, London, where their first two children were born, Joseph Sydney ('Joey', 30 September 1884) and Arthur Annesley Ronald ('Artie' or 'Ronald', 17 January 1886). Ronald Firbank, later a writer and playwright, is perhaps the best known of the family, becoming famous when his writings were posthumously republished in the 1930s. The family moved to the extensive Coopers estate in Chislehurst, Kent, in 1887, where two more children were born, Hubert Somerset ('Bertie', 27 May 1887) and Heather ('Baby' or 'Lassie', 27 August 1888).

In childhood photographs, Heather and her siblings are dressed in stylish though conventional

8 Harriette Firbank in court dress,
photographed by Lafayette Studio, 10 May 1899
V&A: LAFAYETTE ARCHIVE

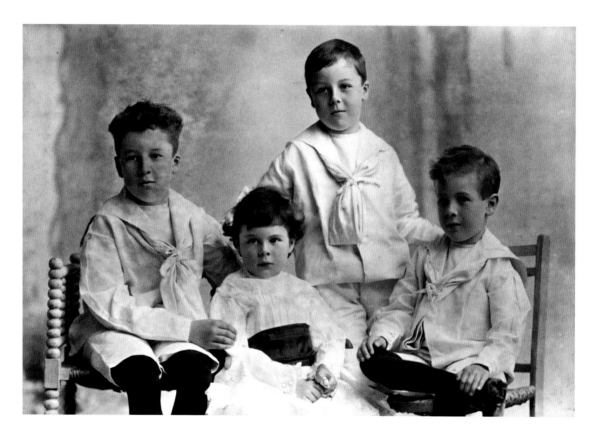

children's clothing [9]. Heather's brothers are seen posed in fashionable sailor suits, while Heather is dressed in a pretty pale frock, with intricate pleating on the front and white floral trim on the sleeves and skirt. Aged around three or four in this picture, Heather would have been used to wearing dresses that were loose around the waist and fashioned from soft fabrics. However, from the age of eight she would have been expected to wear child-sized versions of adult styles, which in the 1890s meant high necklines and full 'leg of mutton' sleeves, although the waist would have remained looser and lower than in women's clothing.[2]

Throughout her life Heather patronized the high-end department store Woolland Brothers of Knightsbridge and it is likely that some of her early clothes were purchased from their well-respected children's department. Alice Keppel, Edward VII's mistress, brought her children down from Edinburgh four times a year to shop at Woollands. Sonia Keppel recalled these visits in her memoirs:

In those days, the 'Juvenile Department' at Woollands was situated on the third or fourth floor. Grimly, the lift man shut his concertina-gates on us, and very, very slowly we ascended to our appointment with 'No. 10'.

We never discovered whether 'No. 10' had had Christian baptism and a name of her own. To Violet and me, she remained a numerical cypher that sucked pins. Always she was bent double at our feet, measuring our skirts, slithering round on her poor, old knees.[3]

During the early years of Heather's life the family owned several properties, including the St Julian's estate in Newport, South Wales (a large manor house rebuilt by Joseph Firbank), as well as the Coopers estate in Kent and smaller, less permanent residences in Mayfair. Her father confirmed his status as a respected man of the upper middle classes when he was elected as Conservative MP for East Hull in 1895.

Heather's brothers were sent to boarding school at a young age, while Heather was tutored at home by her German governess. She became fluent in German, French and Italian, was a gifted pianist [14] and wrote poetry and short stories; she later translated one of her brother Ronald's books into German. However, it seems that it was from her mother, Harriette, a keen collector of *objets d'art* who filled the family homes with paintings, porcelain, ivories and tapestries, that Heather acquired her love of beautiful things [13].

'HOW GOOD GOD HAS BEEN TO US DARLING'
The Firbanks' fortunes were in the ascendant at the turn of the century and in 1902, when Heather was 14, her father was awarded a knighthood in the King's Coronation Honours, in recognition of his successful career as a Conservative politician and as High Sheriff of Monmouthshire.[4] The newly titled Lady Firbank, who attended the coronation along with her family [10], wrote to Heather's brother Ronald in December, 'How good God has been to us darling all through the year now nearly so past.'[5]

Edward VII openly welcomed newly rich industrialists, businessmen and their families into royal

circles. Lady Dorothy Nevill satirized the attitude of the old guard towards this influx of commercial and industrial money into London society: 'The old social privileges of birth and breeding were swept aside by the mob of plebeian wealth which surged into the drawing room, the portals of which had until then been so jealously guarded.'[6] While the Firbanks' wealth was not enough to grant access into the very oldest and highest court circles (the top 1 per cent of British society in 1911–13 comprised a tiny group who owned 69 per cent of the nation's capital),[7] their rise from coal mining to titled elite in just two generations was meteoric. Heather was destined to be a privileged debutante presented at court and was educated in the proper behaviour and social etiquette pertaining to a young woman of her class.

As an adolescent on the brink of womanhood, Heather would have absorbed the Edwardian fashion scene through her women's magazines, a selection of which survive in the V&A's collection. She was not yet old enough to be 'out' in society, so her clothes were made by lesser-known dressmakers, probably to designs chosen by her mother. Although no clothes survive from Heather's early teens, we can build up a picture of what she might have worn through surviving family photographs [11]. Save for a few subtle differences – such as slightly shorter skirts, fewer complicated trimmings and lighter colours – Heather's dresses would have closely resembled her mother's. In the 1900s this meant high necklines, the waist nipped in by a corset at the natural height and the bosom accentuated. Her hair would have been worn long and tied with a ribbon bow.

A letter written to her brother Ronald when Heather was around 15 reveals a little of her adolescent character. She mocks her mother and shows that, like her brother, who later became well known for his writings on the subject, she had an acute awareness of and even a touch of cynicism about the importance placed on keeping up appearances by members of the circles in which she moved. Anticipating the forthcoming family holiday, she writes:

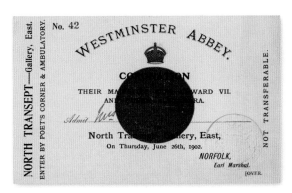

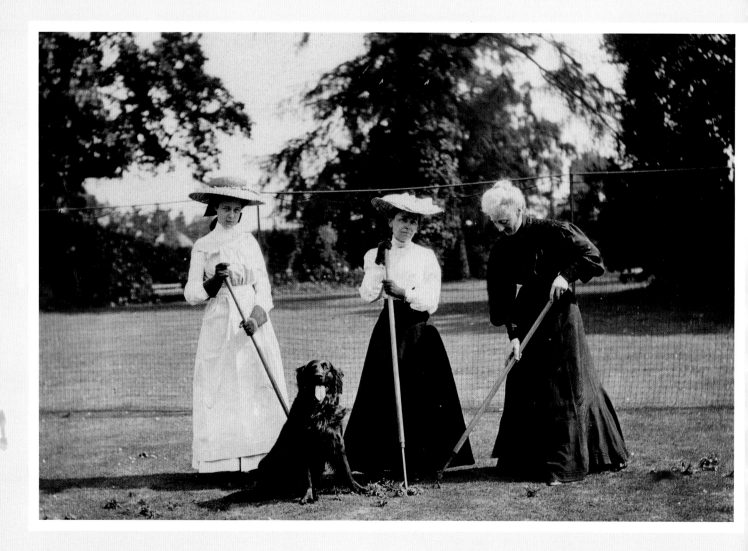

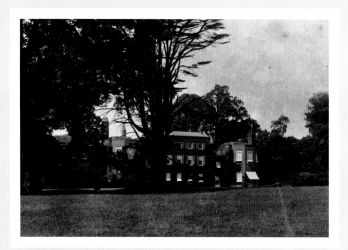

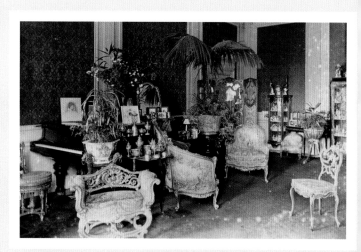

11 *top* In the garden at the Coopers: (from left to right) Heather Firbank aged about 15, unknown woman, Harriette Firbank, *c*.1903

12 *above left* The Coopers, the Firbank family home, Chislehurst, Kent, *c*.1903

13 *above right* Interior of the Coopers, *c*.1904

ALL V&A: HEATHER FIRBANK ARCHIVE

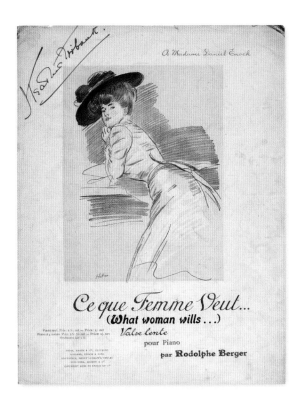

14 *'Ce que Femme Veut ...'* (What woman wills ...),
illustrated cover for Heather's piano sheet music,
Enoch & Sons, Paris, *c.*1905
V&A: HEATHER FIRBANK ARCHIVE

*[S]he always says when we get to the Hotel, 'now
Lassie you must have this room, "yes", (to the door-
man who shows us to the rooms!) My little girl will
have this room!! & my two "youngest"! Boys can
have this, & then my little girls "maid" can have this
room (which is up in the attic!) & then "Sir Thomas"
MP!!! can have this room when he comes, which is so
rare, because he's so busy'!*[8]

Sadly, the Firbank family's good fortune did not last
long. In 1904, serious financial difficulties precipi-
tated a downward spiral that led to Thomas Firbank
being forced to sell the country estate in Chislehurst,
including their mid-eighteenth-century home, the
Coopers [12]. Auction catalogues and photographs
survive which document the comfortable, conventional and luxurious interiors of Heather's childhood
home, which was decorated with late-eighteenth-
century English and French porcelain, furniture and
silver, interspersed with large and fashionable palms
in splendid jardinières [13]. A two-day sale took
place at Christie, Manson and Woods, King Street,
St James's Square, London, in May 1904, which included much of Lady Firbank's art collection.[9] Sir
Thomas Firbank was still Conservative MP for East
Hull and the public humiliation for the couple must
have been extreme. This auction marked an irrevers-
ible turning point in the fortunes and social standing
of the family, making it all the more important for

Heather, the only daughter, to maintain the appropriate appearance for a woman in society.

As her earliest and closest adviser on what to
wear, Lady Firbank would have been the strongest
influence on Heather's clothing choices in her early
adulthood. Fortunately for Heather, her mother was a
highly fashionable woman, well accustomed to luxurious dressing. Photographed by the studio of royal
photographer James Lafayette in 1899, Lady Firbank
appears in a fine court dress with an abundance of
sumptuous fabrics and trimmings, looking confident
and refined [8]. As a member of the aristocracy, Harriette would have understood the importance of her
public image. An extract from one of Ronald's early
pieces, 'Ideas and Fancies', in 1904, provides an astute
observation of this preoccupation. Although he does
not explicitly make his mother his subject, his words
hint at the Firbanks' awareness of their precarious
social position. Accompanied by a sketch of a woman
in an evening gown [15], Ronald's annotation reads:

*Nobody knew quite who she was, nobody had any-
thing exactly against her. One saw her everywhere,
and she was always so beautifully dressed. She said
her husband was 'in business' and everyone admired
her for so cleverly concealing him. She must be all
right people said, or the Duchess would never have
spoken to her.*[10]

The earliest dress in the Heather Firbank Collection dates from about 1905, when Heather was 18.
The dress, which has no label, was probably made
by a lesser-known dressmaker to be worn for an
informal summer occasion such as a boating party
[17]. It is fashioned from lightweight cotton fabric,
with a stylistic nod to nautical clothing in its blue
and white stripes. We are able to date this as the
earliest of Heather's surviving garments as the dress
has a high neck and is formed of a separate bodice
and skirt, as was the norm at the beginning of the
century. (Another slightly later dress of Heather's
made of a separate bodice and skirt but with a flat
collar is kept at the Museum of London.[11]) Around

15 Sketch and notes from 'Ideas and Fancies',
Ronald Firbank, c.1904
COURTESY OF LORD HORDER

16 Petticoat, cotton, trimmed with machine embroidery,
machine lace and silk ribbon, British, c.1906
V&A: T.67–1960

17 Summer day dress, cotton trimmed with broderie
anglaise, machine lace and pearl buttons, British, c.1905
V&A: T.21A-C–1960

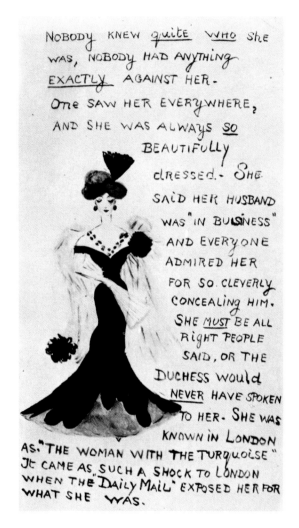

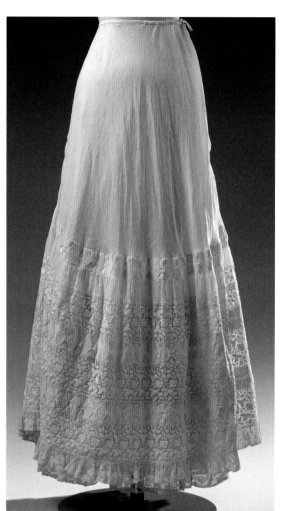

1907–8 bodices and skirts became joined at the waist and all of the later surviving day and evening dresses are made in this way. The shape of the boating dress is also in keeping with the mid-Edwardian fashion for a small waist and voluminous bosom. The bodice closes at the back with a row of hooks and eyes and is made of several panels of fabric pulled in at the 'V'-shaped waistband to create volume at the front, while a wide self-fabric belt covers the join at the waist. There is no boning in the bodice, but the fashionable high lace neckpiece is reinforced by five metal supports and closes tightly at the back with

hooks and eyes. The skirt of the dress is pleated and would have been worn with a petticoat to add to its fullness. A beautifully intricate white cotton petticoat trimmed with pink ribbon shows how weight and volume were achieved with multiple layers of fabric and heavy trimmings [**16**].

As she prepared to 'come out' as a society woman, Heather's interest in fashion intensified. From 1908 the collection contains fashion plates and press drawings almost obsessively cut out and kept from newspapers and women's magazines, including numerous illustrations by Bessie Ascough from the women's

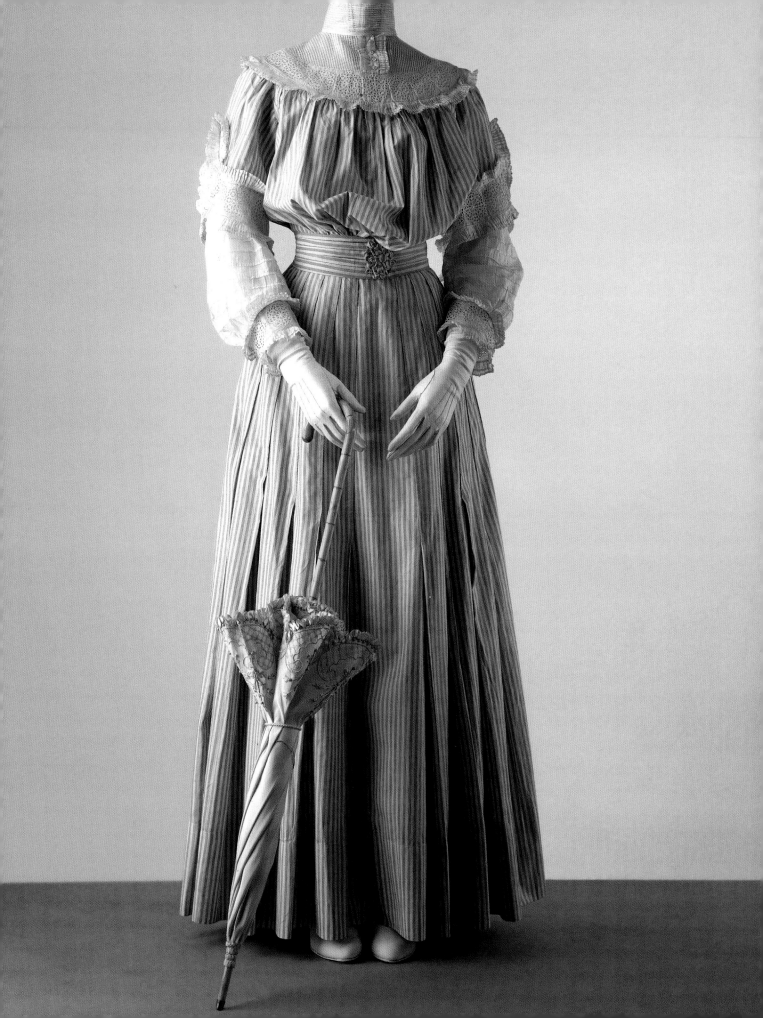

18 'Dress of "Tuxedo" cloth sketched at Mme. Elizabeth's', illustrated by W. Brooke Alder, cutting from *Country Life*, 16 May 1908, with annotations by Heather Firbank

V&A: HEATHER FIRBANK ARCHIVE

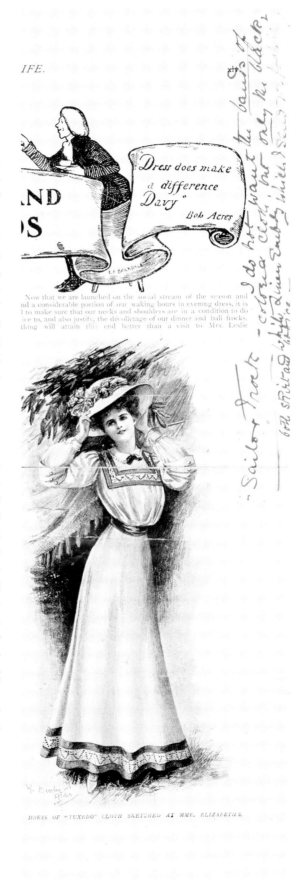

IFE.

Dress does make
a difference
Davy"
Bob Acres

Now that we are launched on the social stream of the season and
nd a considerable portion of our waking hours in evening dress, it is
l to make sure that our necks and shoulders are in a condition to do
ce to, and also justify, the decolletage of our dinner and ball frocks,
thing will attain this end better than a visit to Mrs. Leslie

DRESS OF "TUXEDO" CLOTH SKETCHED AT MME. ELIZABETH'S.

pages of daily newspapers, such as 'For and About Women' from the *Evening Standard and St James's Gazette*, 'Of Interest to Women' from the *Daily Mail* and features from periodicals such as *The Queen*, *Sketch* and *Tatler*, among others. Heather used the images as direct inspiration for her clothing choices. Several correspond closely to dresses which survive, and one from *Country Life*, 16 May 1908, which is annotated with instructions to the dressmaker, clearly shows her detailed involvement in the designs for the clothes that she wore. It reads, 'Sailor Frock I do not want the bands of colored cloth, but only the black & white linen emdby [embroidery] which I send you for trimming both skirt and bodice' [18].

'AN EPOCH IN A WOMAN'S LIFE':
PRESENTATION AT COURT

Formal presentation to royalty at court, which continued up until 1958, was a rite of passage and a celebration of a young woman's initiation into the adult world. It also acted as a filter to maintain the exclusivity of the upper classes. A young woman was only permitted to be presented and to enter the privileged world of society events, parties and balls – where, importantly, it was hoped that she would meet her future husband – if she was sponsored by an established member of society who had been presented at court herself. For Heather, who was sponsored by her mother, this ceremonial acceptance ushered her into womanhood and validated her position among the upper classes.

Noting the central importance of court presentation in a debutante's young life, a journalist in *Harmsworth Magazine* in 1900 stressed:

Presentation at Court is an epoch in a woman's life not easily forgotten. To a young girl it signifies a transition from girlhood to womanhood; from the obscurity of the schoolroom to the brilliancy of Society life, in which at homes, dinners, balls, garden parties, operas and theatres follow each other in a continuous whirl.[12]

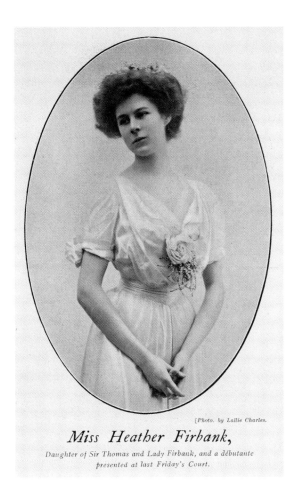

[Photo. by Lallie Charles.]

Miss Heather Firbank,

Daughter of Sir Thomas and Lady Firbank, and a débutante presented at last Friday's Court.

1908: HEATHER'S DEBUT

Heather's presentation at court at the age of 20 (two years older than the norm) allowed her to begin attending society functions and events as a debutante. The preparations for a young woman's debut could last for months. Cynthia Asquith, the debutante daughter of the 11th Earl of Wemyss, born in the same year as Heather, remembered it as 'weeks busied with long lessons in deportment ... panic-stricken rehearsals of my curtsey' and 'endless wearisome hours of trying-on'.[13] The day involved lengthy queues, but the ceremony itself lasted only minutes, with each debutante taking her turn to curtsey at the feet of the seated king and queen. After the ceremonies, accounts of the events were provided in ladies' magazines and society columns in newspapers, where notable debutantes were singled out for a full description of their clothing.

For the Firbank family, it was vital that their only daughter make the right impression on this most public of occasions, and nothing but the very best was acceptable. From their house in fashionable Mayfair, perfectly positioned to visit London's finest tailors and court dressmakers, Heather and her mother would have made numerous shopping trips to prepare her wardrobe in the weeks leading up to the ceremony, attending numerous fittings for her presentation gown at one of the many London fashion houses describing themselves as 'court dressmakers'. The dress would have been custom-made, albeit with an effort to adhere to the rules of that particular year as prescribed by the Lord Chamberlain's Office. These rules dictated hem length, suitable materials and colour (always white or cream), headwear and, very importantly, the length of the court train, an additional sumptuous panel of silk, often embroidered and padded, which was attached at the shoulders of the gown and extended behind the wearer. In the Edwardian period the court train was reaching its zenith in both size and extravagance: for 1908, a length of between 3 and 4 yards (2.7 and 3.6 metres) was standard.[14]

Although her presentation gown does not survive, the society magazine *The Onlooker* featured a photograph of Heather in her finery, along with a pearl headdress fixed on a fashionably wide hairstyle with a decorative tulle and heather trimming on her chest [19]. The description reads, 'Miss Firbank ... made the prettiest picture in a Princesse frock of crêpe de chine embroidered with pearls and crystals, while her train of satin was lightly trimmed with tulle ruchings caught here and there with sprays of white heather, her name flower.'[15]

'IT IS SO NICE TO BE NOTED FOR SOMETHING': BUILDING AN IMAGE

Although Heather was dressed fashionably before her coming out, her restricted social life as an adolescent would not have been public enough to warrant the high-status clothes of well-known dressmakers. Once a young woman had debuted, however, there followed a whirl of social events known as 'the season', which ran from April to August and included annual sporting events such as the Henley Regatta and racing at Royal Ascot, artistic events such as the

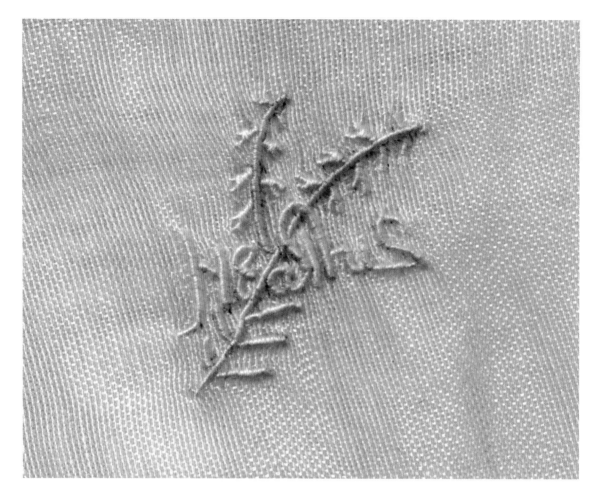

opening of the Royal Academy Summer Exhibition, and a round of dinner parties, garden parties and balls, evocatively described in Vita Sackville-West's observational novel *The Edwardians* (1930):

the pageant of the Season, the full exciting existence in London, the crowds, the colour, the hot streets by day, the cool balconies at night, the flowers filling the rooms and the flower-girls with baskets at the street corners, the endless parties with people streaming in and out of doors and up and down the stairs; the display, the luxury, the wealth, the elegance ... [16]

Photography also played an important part in building a public image and Heather made several trips to photographers' studios to have her portrait taken. These photographs acted as publicity shots or calling cards and could be provided at a moment's notice should a magazine or newspaper want to feature the young 'deb'. The V&A has three photographs of Heather from about 1909 taken by the fashionable society photographer Baron de Meyer, who later worked for *Vogue*, *Vanity Fair* and *Harper's Bazaar* [21]. Photographer Cecil Beaton, who cites

de Meyer as one of his key inspirations, described him as 'a great snob ... if he photographed a certain woman, the implication was that she had attained a high position in the social scene'.[17] A number of studio portraits by Lallie Charles, dating from about 1908, also survive, one of which was chosen to accompany the description of Heather in *The Onlooker*. Several show her posed alongside bunches of heather, which was used as a personal trademark for the young Miss Firbank, with the heather motif occurring again and again on headed paper, Christmas cards and even a pair of her drawers, which were embroidered with her slanting signature written through a sprig of the plant [20]. This association was secured further by the numerous clothes in her wardrobe fashioned in heather colours, ranging from deep purple to pale mauve. Although it is true that such colours were fashionable at the time – the etiquette of mourning dress stipulated that purple was an appropriate colour for half-mourning – it was also conceivably part of Heather's campaign to create a memorable and unique self-image to help distinguish her from the crowd.

Two works by Heather's brother Ronald under-line the obsessive need to be memorable in society circles. In the short story 'A Study in Temperament', published in 1905, the protagonist, Lady Agnes, is described as being 'noted for having the most beauti-ful hair in London'. The importance of this is high-lighted by the comment, 'It is so nice to be noted for something.'[18] The parallel with Heather's experience is even clearer in Ronald's short play 'A Disciple from the Country', in which we read that 'Mrs Creamway, a rich Australian widow, is launching her daughter Stella in London Society ... Stella's "line" is to be ultra-*dévote*, in consequence of which she is known in Society as "Saint Angelica"'.[19]

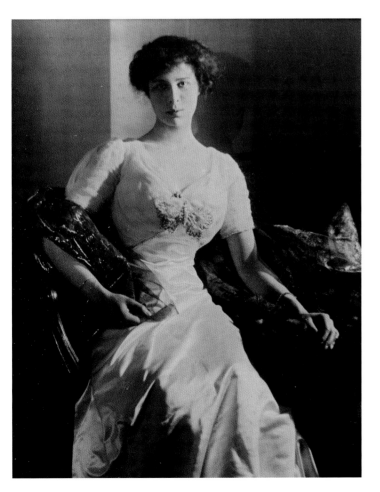

As Ronald had such a close relationship with his mother and sister, it seems inevitable that he took inspiration for his writings from their lives and concerns. Heather's 'line', it seems, was to be dis-tinguished by her wearing of purple and frequent associations with the heather flower, a theme which continued through her early twenties and is seen in some of the most iconic pieces in her wardrobe [see **36** and **83**, for example].

It was drummed into a young debutante that it was her duty to her family, their friends and her social class to conform to all the rules of sartorial etiquette – the correct tilt of the hat, management of flowing skirts and length of gloves – and to do so with mod-esty, dignity, charm and style. Mrs Humphry, a writer of etiquette guides in the late nineteenth and early twentieth centuries, declared firmly in 1897:

One can almost invariably distinguish the well-bred
girl at the first glance, whether she is walking, shop-
ping, in an omnibus, descending from a carriage
or a cab, or sauntering up and down in the park.
There is a quiet self-possession about the gentle-
woman, whether young or old, that marks her
out from women of a lower class, whose manner
is florid.[20]

Born into privilege and great wealth, Heather Firbank was positioned from early on to be a 'lady of fashion', shaping her public image through clothes and photography. As an only daughter, a symbolic rather than an active anchor of the Firbank family's status, this image was important for all of them. The roots of her highly fashionable wardrobe, her love of fashion and her expectations in life were established in these early years.

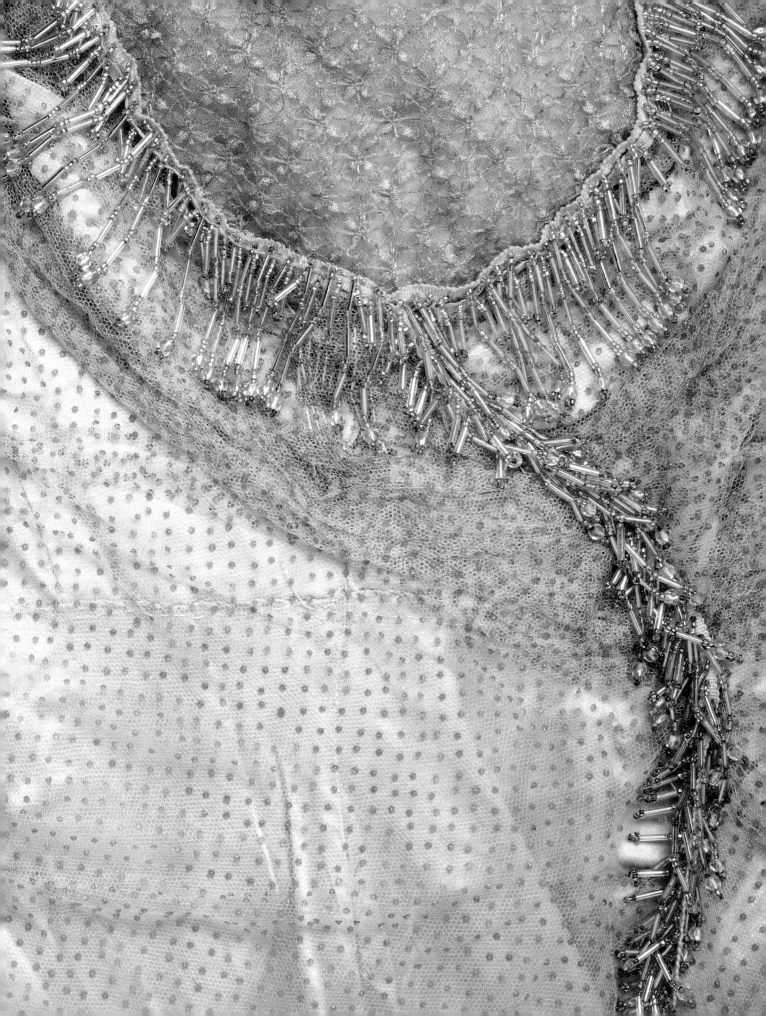

THE SOCIAL WHIRL:
A SOCIETY WARDROBE FOR THE SEASON
1908–10

In 1908, the Firbanks divided their time between their house at 11 Hill Street, Mayfair, where they were supported by 16 members of staff,[1] and a rented property called Newlands on the Petworth estate in rural Sussex. Having come out, Heather was now able to take her place in London society as a new debutante. Life among the aristocracy and upper middle classes followed a seasonal cycle related to traditional royal court practice. In addition to annual artistic and sporting events such as the opening of the Royal Academy Summer Exhibition, Henley Regatta and Royal Ascot that have already been mentioned, there could be as many as three balls a night during the season and attendance was all but obligatory.

DRESSING FOR OCCASION

Dress played an essential role in all this activity. For each different event there was a specific style and type of garment to be worn and it was crucial that these showed an awareness of current trends and changes in fashion. For example, one of the most important changes at this time, as clearly reflected in Heather's wardrobe, was the introduction of the straighter, more natural silhouette known as the 'Directoire' line [23, and see page 1]. Although part of a general move towards a new shape, the French designer Paul Poiret claimed that he had invented this more upright look; but while it appeared less constricting and artificial, and the designer declared that he had 'freed the bust', the smooth line was still orchestrated from beneath with corsetry.

Heather's surviving underwear reveals how this was achieved. Her corset (or pair of corsets, as they were referred to at the time), made from fine cream silk and purple braid, worn over a simple chemise and bloomers, was positioned under the bust and reached down almost to the top of the thighs [26]. This pulled in the waist and smoothed the hips to provide the sleek, straight line required. From about 1905, suspenders were attached to corsets and these would have held up her stockings [25], replacing the earlier need for a suspender belt or garters. A bust bodice, a small ruched silk garment which covered the top of the chest above where the corset began, would sometimes have been worn over the corset for added protection and modesty. A precursor to the modern brassiere, two lilac satin examples of bust bodices survive in Heather's wardrobe.

Keeping up appearances was a day-long occupation, involving several changes of clothes and an extensive wardrobe. From first thing in the morning, when she got out of bed in her delicate *saut du lit* (morning robe), to changing into her tailored morning costume for shopping or sports, then into a formal afternoon dress for visiting, before returning to put on a loose tea gown, then donning a formal evening dress for dinner and finally dressing for the grandest of balls and court presentations, a society woman was constantly judged on how she looked. Among the wealthy and fashionable, it was not just garments that were seasonally styled, but also hats and accessories, each requiring summer, winter, town and country versions.

In a 1913 article entitled 'The Secret of Smart Dressing' in the monthly general-interest magazine *The Strand*, Gordon Meggy (advised by Lady Duff-Gordon, who styled her Lucile dresses for the accompanying photographs and took a 'personal interest' in the preparation of the article), suggested:

22 Ball dress (detail of plate 49)

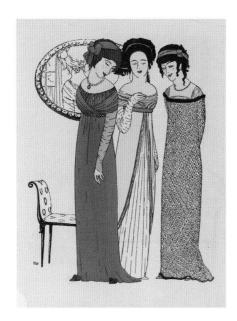

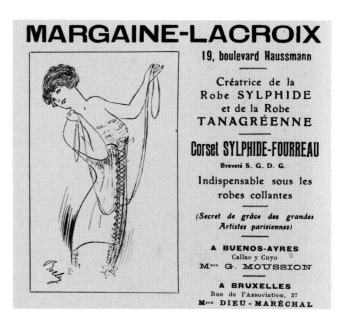

23 *above left* Fashion plate from *Les Robes de Paul Poiret*, Paul Iribe, Paris, 1908
V&A: NAL

24 *above right* Advertisement for Margaine-Lacroix from *Les Modes*, Paris, August 1910
V&A: HEATHER FIRBANK ARCHIVE

25 *below* Group of single stockings (from left to right): cotton lisle, England *c.*1908, wool 'Balbriggan' with embroidered clocks, Ireland, *c.*1912, machine-knitted silk with embroidered clocks, England, *c.*1910, silk, 'Le Cid', France, *c.*1920, wool with openwork detail, England, 1900–1920, wool with embroidered spots, England *c.*1910
V&A: T.95–1960, T.92–1960, T.87–1960, T.85–1960, T.86–1960, T.91–1960

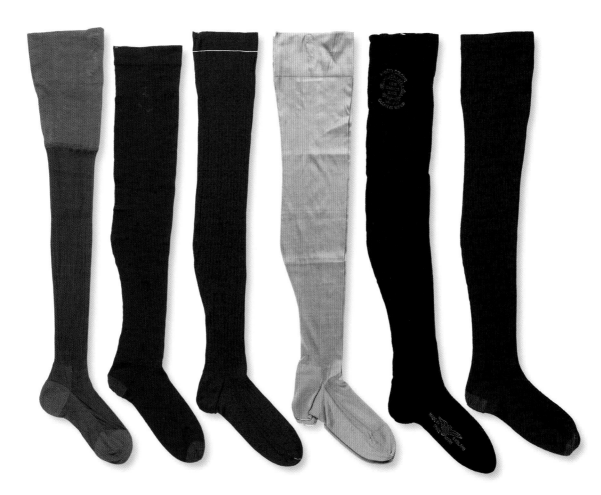

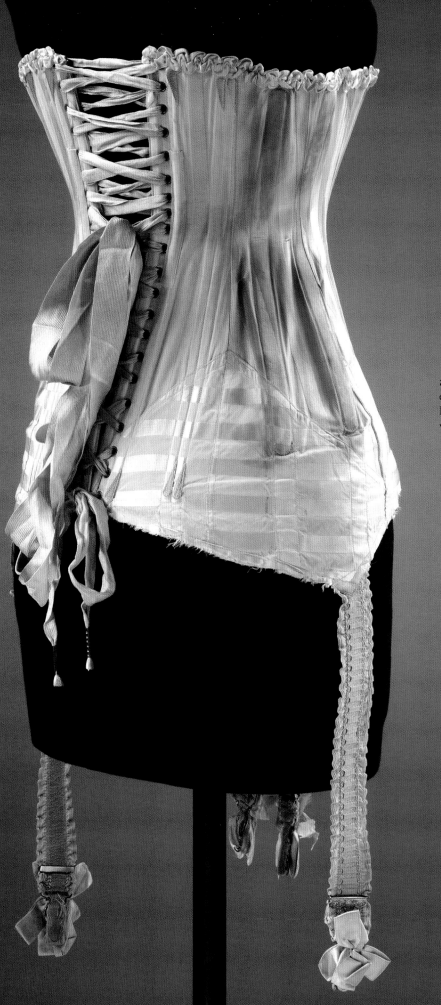

26 Corset, silk with silk ribbon lacings,
elasticated suspenders and metal boning,
London, c.1908
V&A: T.53-1960

The smartest woman is she who is always dressed for the occasion. Whether she is in her motor, walking in the street, travelling, going out to lunch, entertaining friends to tea, or visiting the theatre, she must, in each case, be dressed 'for the part'. It is not simply a question of possessing many different frocks and putting them on in turn to show what a lot of money she spends on dress. Each must be in perfect keeping with the purpose for which it is intended.[2]

For example, the reader is told that 'plain tailor-made dresses are what should be worn in the street', where a woman should never attract 'undue attention' to herself. These should be paired with small plain hats: 'Aigrettes or elaborate plumes of any kind would never, in any circumstances, be worn with a tailor-made dress by a woman who knew what smartness meant.' And diamonds should never be worn in the daytime.

A woman in court society, whether in public or domestic space, was monitored first by her personal maid and then by her family, other household servants, visitors and other women met out shopping, at tea parties and at grand soirées, whether in town or in the country, at home or abroad. Lady Duff-Gordon, one of Heather's favourite dressmakers and proprietor of the exclusive fashion house Lucile, noted in her memoirs how important it was for women of the time to get their 'look' right and how important her role was in achieving this:

I began to be noted for 'making personalities', and the new rich used to come secretly to me to be coached, not only in the art of dressing, but in the art of wearing beautiful clothes, which was far more important for them to acquire ... With all these women I knew that there was only one thing to do, and that was to find them one special 'genre', which they could keep to in their dress and everything which they surrounded themselves. They used to put themselves in my hands absolutely ... I seldom had a failure.[3]

When in the presence of royalty, the need to be dressed according to the last etiquette-correct details,

which had changed little since late Victorian days, was paramount. The wealthiest women in London society dealt with the high demands of their royal court appearances by dressing at the famous and more costly Paris couturiers. They were thus obliged to spend weeks in Paris each year, choosing the required court dresses and fabrics and attending fittings. In April 1904, on one of her annual visits to order her clothes for the forthcoming season, Daisy, Princess of Pless, noted in her diary on 28 April: 'I spent a week in Paris fussing about clothes and left with everything half-finished as I did not want to remain there alone and my little mother left two days after we arrived.'[4] Heather, however, did not order her wardrobe from Paris. This may have been purely a personal preference, but as a single woman it would not have been as easy for her to make trips abroad. For many wealthy women their entrée to Parisian circles came through their husbands, whom they accompanied on their travels. As she never married, Heather did not have the same ease of access to this world. She could have travelled with her brother or mother as chaperone, but it seems that she preferred instead to shop at the very best retailers that London had to offer, and she did so alongside some of the smartest and best-dressed society women.

Stories of faux pas made by women who had failed to dress correctly circulated around society groups, acting as cautionary tales for the ingénue debutante. Margot Tennant (later Asquith, Countess of Oxford), daughter of Charles Clow Tennant, industrialist and politician, was a debutante in the mid-1880s. One evening, when already out to dinner, she received an urgent late summons from her father to a royal reception at the home of Lord Randolph Churchill, where the Prince of Wales was to be present. She went dressed as she was – in her dinner dress – 'a white muslin dress with transparent chemise sleeves, a fichu and a long skirt with a Nattier blue taffeta sash'. As soon as she entered the room she realized that all the women were in full court evening dress. 'All the fine ladies [were] wearing ball-dresses off the

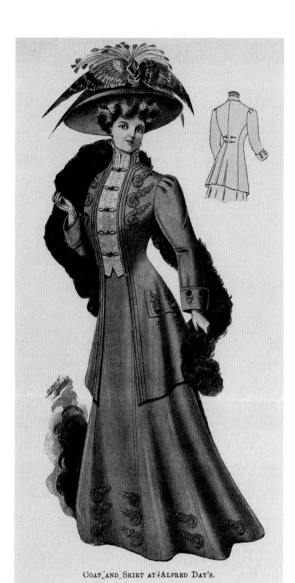

27 'Coat and skirt at Alfred Day's', cutting from *The Queen*, September 1908
V&A: HEATHER FIRBANK ARCHIVE

COAT AND SKIRT AT ALFRED DAY'S.

DRESSING FOR DAYTIME

The collection of Edwardian day dresses at the V&A is dominated by examples from Heather's wardrobe, including a pink linen summer dress dating from about 1908. Unlike the earlier blue-and-white striped dress, it is formed of a joined bodice and skirt, with two layers of multiple hooks and eyes for fastening at the back and an insert imitating a separate blouse of machine lace and machine-embroidered net. A black velvet ribbon forms a tie at the neck [28]. Day dresses became increasingly simplified in construction and decoration in this period and later examples in Heather's wardrobe – including two straighter, less fussy day dresses by Mascotte – show how they prefigured the increasing simplicity of modern dress. The subtle differences in these Mascotte dresses, one made of silk chiffon and one of wool serge, further highlight the nuances of dressing for different seasons [29, 30].

THE TAILOR-MADE

A distinction was also made between town and country. Heather's life in Mayfair required a town wardrobe, the staple of which was the 'tailor-made' or 'costume' of a jacket and skirt worn with a blouse. For morning and afternoon activities such as shopping, these costumes could make an impact as powerful – though more understated – as luxurious evening wear. Initially based on the tailored riding habits made by male tailors, tailor-mades were established as fashionable daywear for women by Princess Alexandra in the 1880s.

The large number and wide range of designs owned by Heather demonstrate just how important tailored costumes were in a woman's wardrobe. Among them are elegantly tailored jackets and skirts, appropriate for appointments in London, made out of beautiful fine wool serge for spring and autumn and thicker mohair for winter, and sometimes with striking coloured or striped silk linings. Made by the very best London tailors, they include six Redfern tailor-mades and others by Frederick Bosworth, and

shoulder and their tiaras.' She overheard their comments: 'Do look at Miss Tennant! She is in her night gown.' Another remarked, 'I dare say no one told her that the Prince of Wales was coming ... Poor child! What a shame.' The young debutante later wrote in her diary, 'I wished profoundly that I had changed into something smarter before going out.'[5]

As stories like this reveal, there were crucial differences between what was to be worn at different times of day to make the correct impression. One of the remarkable things about the Heather Firbank Collection is that so many different garments survive, allowing us to track the elaborate daily timetable of dressing in this period.

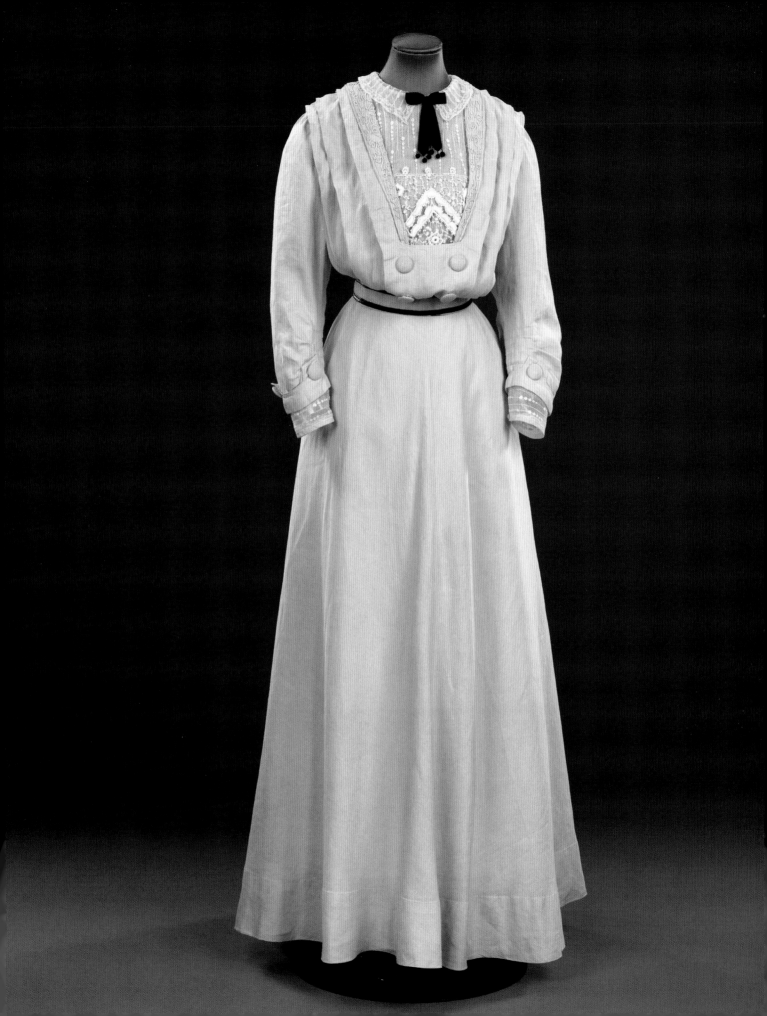

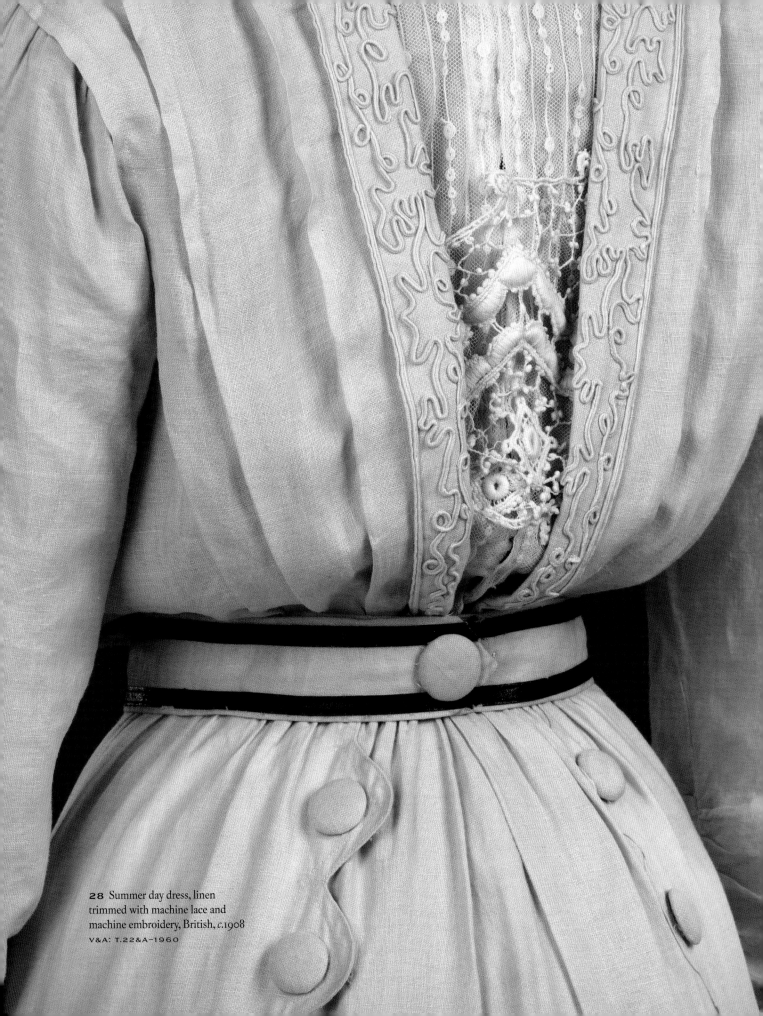

28 Summer day dress, linen trimmed with machine lace and machine embroidery, British, c.1908
V&A: T.22&A-1960

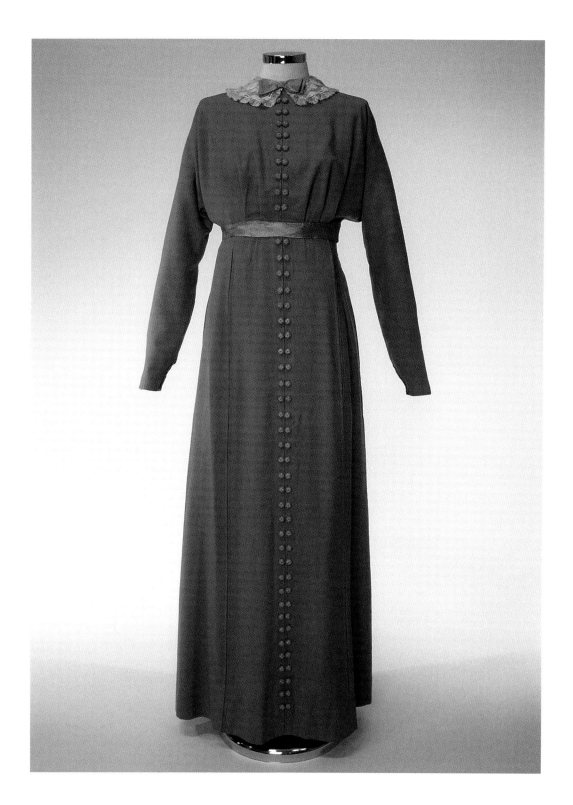

29 Day dress, wool serge trimmed with ribbon
and machine lace collar, Mascotte, London, *c*.1912
GALLERY OF COSTUME, MANCHESTER:
1963.302

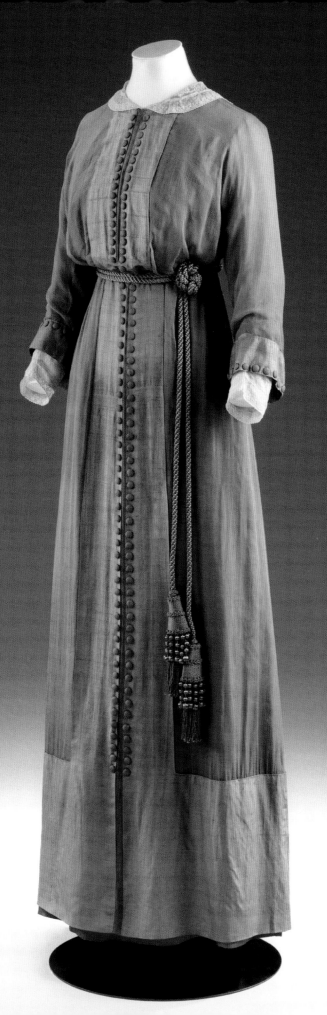

30 Day dress, silk chiffon over silk, with trimmings of machine whitework embroidery, machine lace, silk cord, Mascotte, London, *c*.1912
V&A: CIRC.643-1964

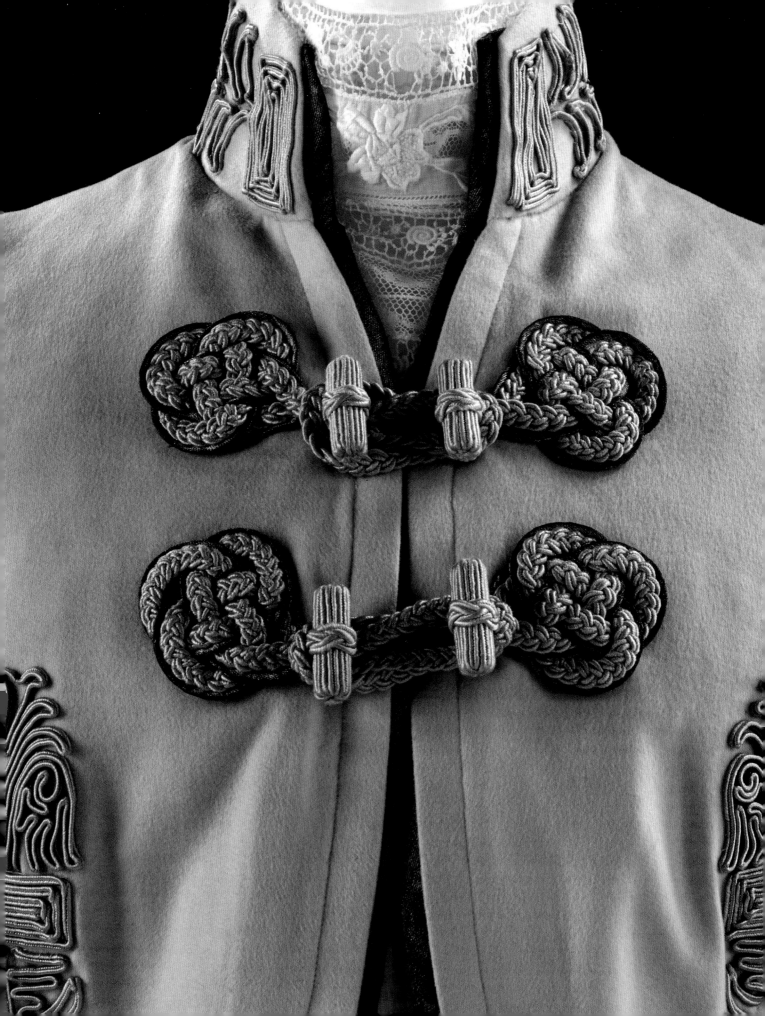

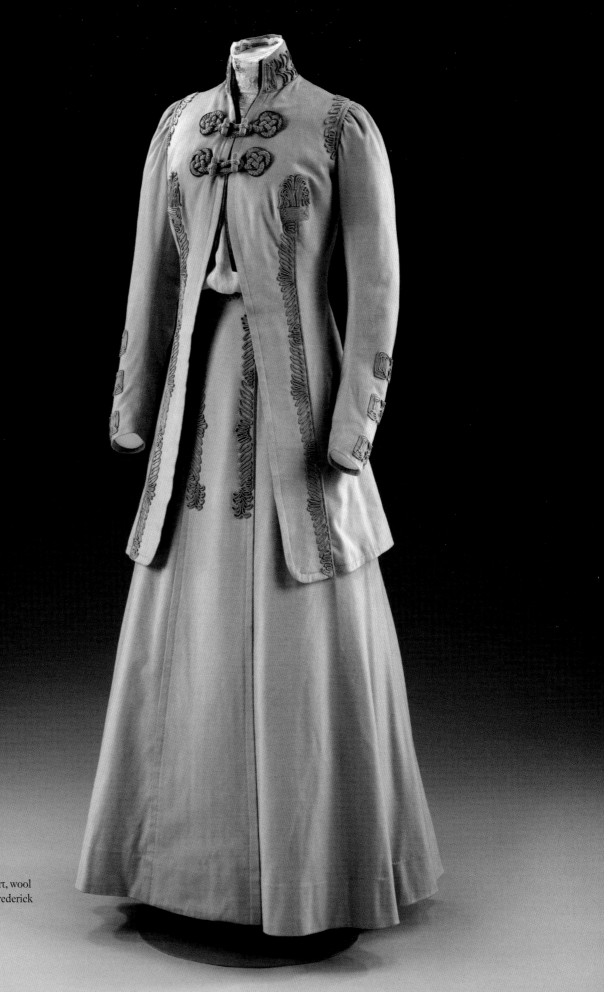

31 Tailored jacket and skirt, wool trimmed with silk braid, Frederick Bosworth, London, c.1908
V&A: T.26&A-1960

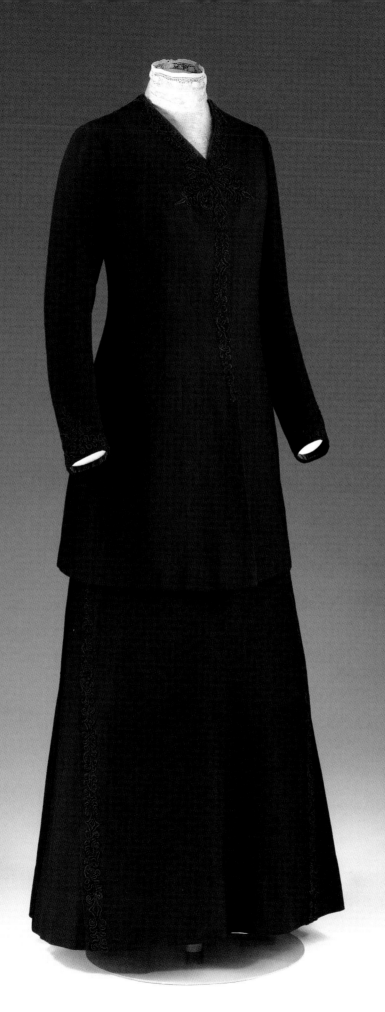

32 Tailored jacket and skirt, wool serge trimmed with silk braid, Redfern, London, *c*.1908

33 Redfern, 26 & 27 Conduit Street and 27 New Bond Street, London, 10 September 1894
ENGLISH HERITAGE

34 Label inside black velvet tailored jacket, woven silk, Redfern, 1909
The coats of arms represent the royal families of Great Britain, Russia and Denmark.
V&A: T.42–1960

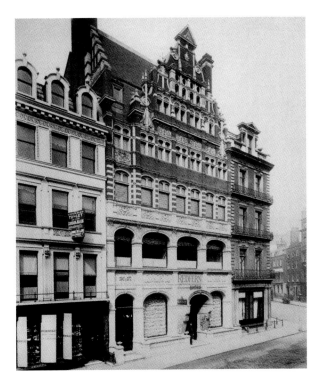

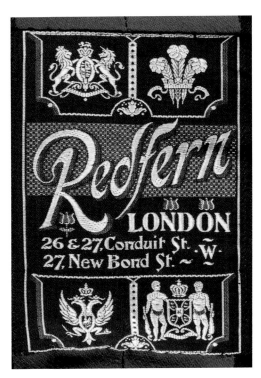

tailors working for the dressmakers Mascotte and Lucile. They exemplify the excellent tailoring London was renowned for in Europe and America.

REDFERN

Heather's favourite tailor was Redfern [**33**]. The company John Redfern & Sons became the world leader in women's tailoring in the nineteenth and early twentieth centuries. Like other specialist tailors, the company expanded its business to include all aspects of fashionable clothing, including court dress.[6] The founder was one of the first to see the fashion potential of the tailor-made and became well known in Paris, as Heather's copies of the Parisian magazine *Les Modes* confirm. Susan North's research published in *Costume* has shown how the company began as a drapery shop in Cowes on the Isle of Wight in the 1840s, where it benefited from the patronage of Queen Victoria and her household at Osborne, and adapted to supply specialist

clothing for sports and events such as the Cowes Regatta. The business operated purely from Cowes High Street until 1876, when a branch opened in Cheshunt, Hertfordshire. This was probably because John Redfern's son (another John) married a Margaret Mims of Cheshunt in 1878. Her brother Frederick Bosworth Mims was a tailor, who managed a new London branch of the business at 26 Conduit Street, off New Bond Street, from 1878. Frederick Bosworth Mims later set up his own independent tailoring and court-dressmaking business at 9 New Burlington Street, between Regent Street and Savile Row, in 1903, trading there until 1913. He provided Heather with her tweed golf costume [see **69**] and a lavender-grey (now faded) wool tailored jacket and skirt with twisting braid [**31**], as well as a 'white flannel coat and skirt trimmed with braid'.[7] An example of a miniature afternoon outfit and hat bearing a Frederick Bosworth label can be seen on a doll in the V&A collections.[8]

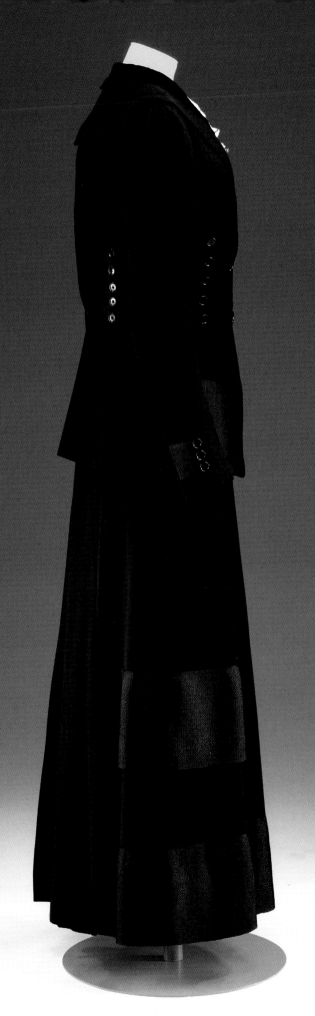

35 Tailored jacket and skirt, wool serge
with velvet collar and jacquard woven
silk braid, Redfern, London, *c.*1911
V&A: CIRC.647&A-1964

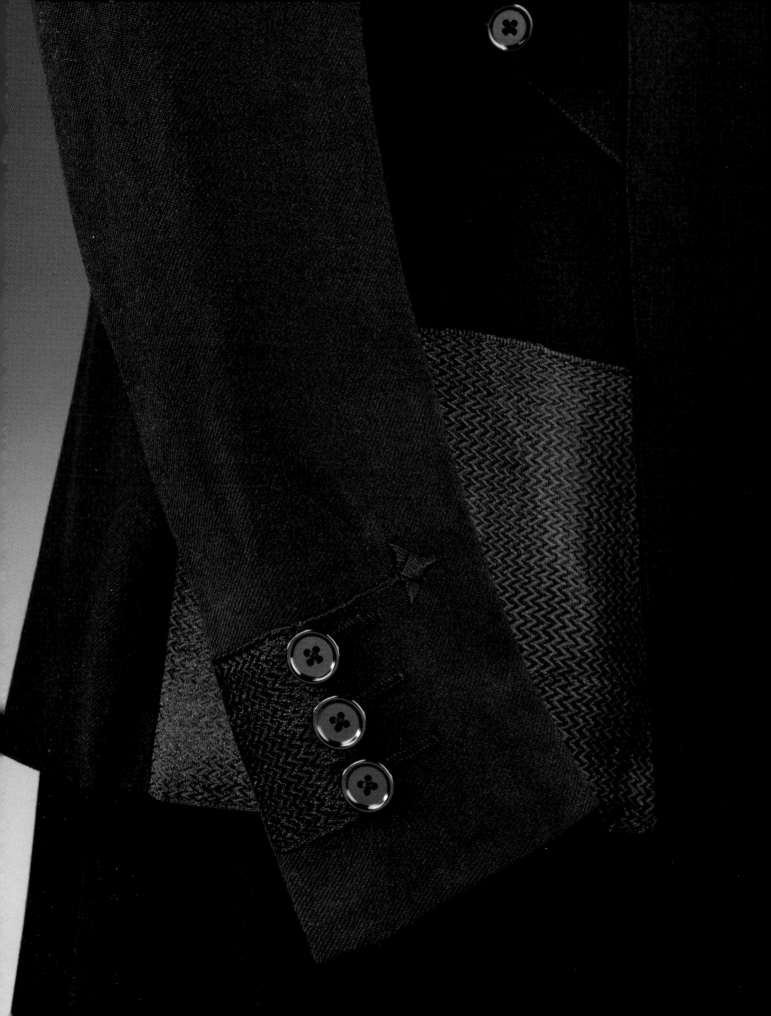

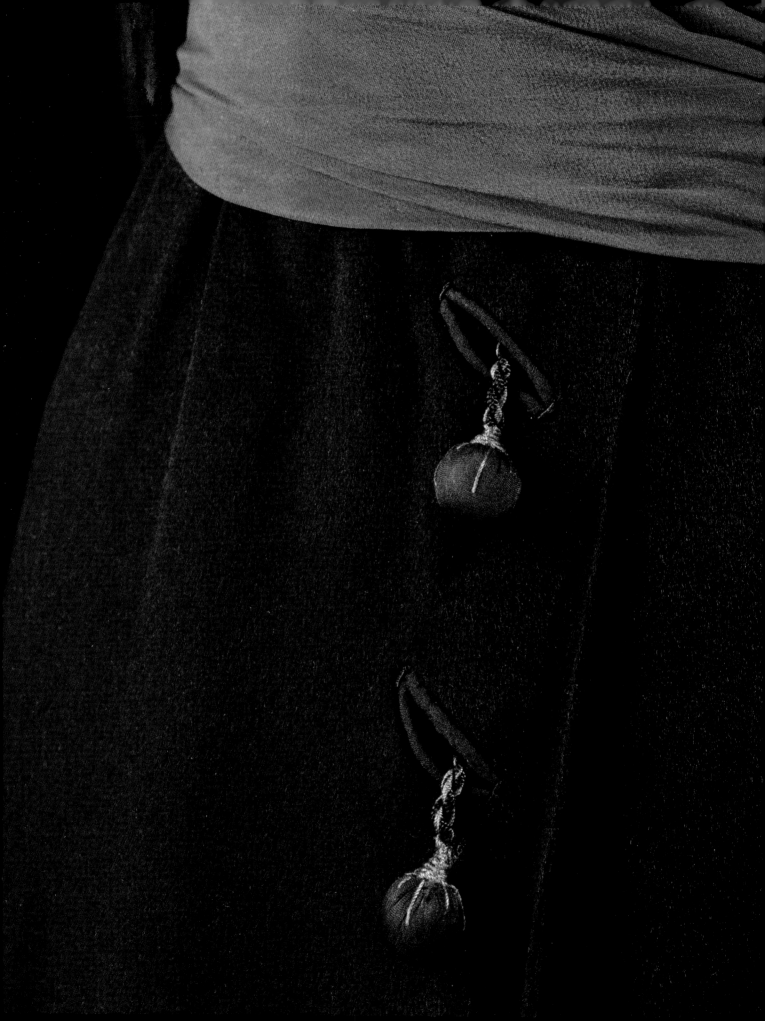

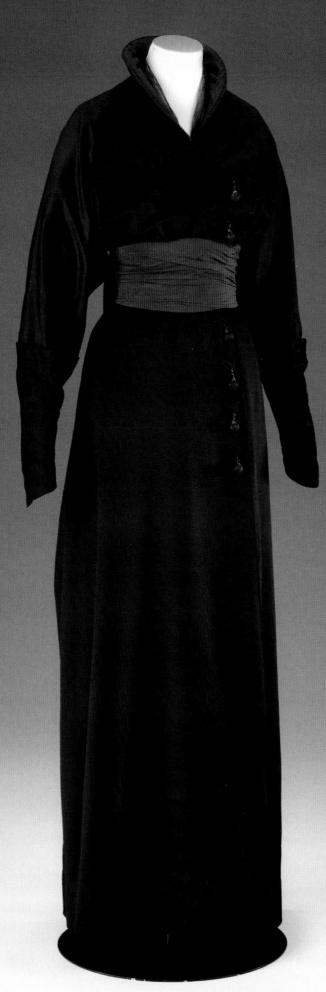

36 Afternoon dress, cashmere
trimmed with silk crêpe, Redfern,
London, *c.*1913
V&A: T.32–1960

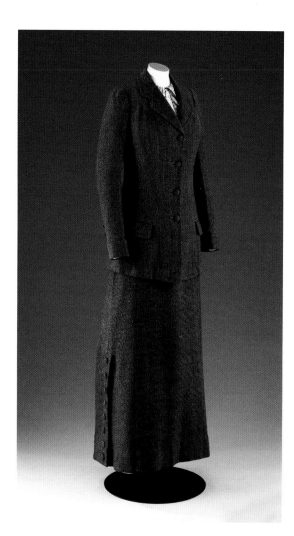

37 Tailored jacket and skirt, woollen tweed, Redfern, London, c.1911
V&A: T.28&A-1960

38 Blouse, cotton with machine lace inserts and hand-worked embroidery, British, c.1908
V&A: T.59-1960

example, dating from about 1908, is of fine-quality navy-blue serge (a twill-woven woollen cloth widely used in women's tailoring) and is trimmed with black at the collar, closing edges and cuffs. The gently flared skirt is decorated in the same way, emphasizing the feminine fluted silhouette, which recalls the fluid lines of Art Nouveau. Both costumes have flared gored skirts, which would have been paired with decorative, feminine, high-necked blouses to provide a detailed counterpoint to this otherwise sober combination.

Heather's tailor-made costumes became increasingly restrained as each year went by, relying on cut and quality of fabric to achieve a strong visual impact. One example from about 1909 is plain and undecorated, fastening with a single covered button, but made of luxurious black silk velvet and lined with a surprising bright blue and black striped silk [**34**]. Redfern also created a less formal tailor-made costume for Heather of diagonally striped black and grey wool tweed [**37**] cut with simple revers at the collar and trimmed only with covered buttons at the side seams of the skirt. These emphasize the increasingly vertical silhouette and help to date the costume to about 1911. It was probably made for town wear, because of its dark, businesslike colour, although its understated style suggests that it was suitable for everyday dress or for travelling in winter.

Two of Heather's Redfern tailor-made costumes reflect the strong movement towards borrowing masculine styles in the years leading up to the First World War. A dark grey serge example of about 1912 is double-breasted, fastens with uncompromising plain buttons and a buttoning belt, has contrasting collar and cuffs of black silk velvet, and has a very plain skirt with a turned-up hem – perhaps a witty reference to the turn-ups on men's trousers.[9] A tailor-made dating from about 1911, finished with a sailor-style collar and using a range of trimmings emulating masculine styles, has a shorter hemline. This exhibits a range of subtle contrasts between textures: navy-blue velvet against black serge, black

Redfern was an international operation, with branches opening in Paris in 1881 (242 rue de Rivoli) and New York in 1884 (210 Fifth Avenue and 1132 Broadway). Heather was a regular London customer from 1909 until 1914, when the business traded from 26 & 27 Conduit Street, which was connected with 27 New Bond Street, as a surviving bill shows [see **112**]. The company's London base remained at Conduit Street for over 40 years, from 1878 until 1922. Heather's Redfern tailor-made costumes come from a period when the company was a serious rival to the leading Paris couturier, British-born Charles Frederick Worth. The house of Redfern operated on a different business model to that of Worth, employing other in-house designers, opening a total of 11 branches to increase access to customers, and advertising extensively in magazines including *The Queen*.

Two of Heather's tailored costumes – one by Redfern [**32**] and one by Frederick Bosworth [**31**] – have jackets decorated with sinuous trails of braid reminiscent of military frogging. The Redfern

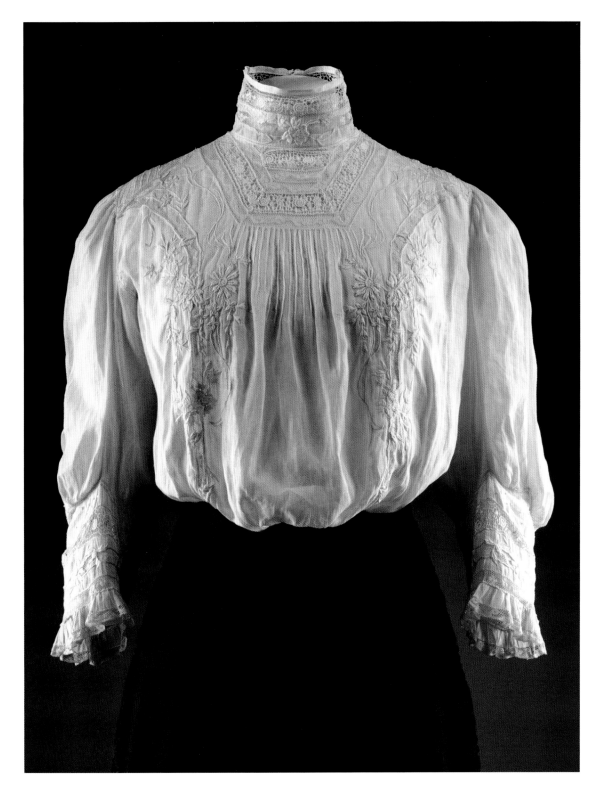

horn buttons, bands of glossy woven silk braid, and hand-stitched buttonholes, some of the functioning ones given extra definition with intricate binding of navy-blue satin, and cuffs finished with hand-worked arrowheads [35]. This tailor-made costume displays an impressive attention to detail and affirms the creativity of the designers and the skills of the tailors employed at Redfern.

The Heather Firbank Collection also includes two Redfern dresses, which would have been made in a separate dressmaking workroom and show the range of their products beyond the tailor-mades on

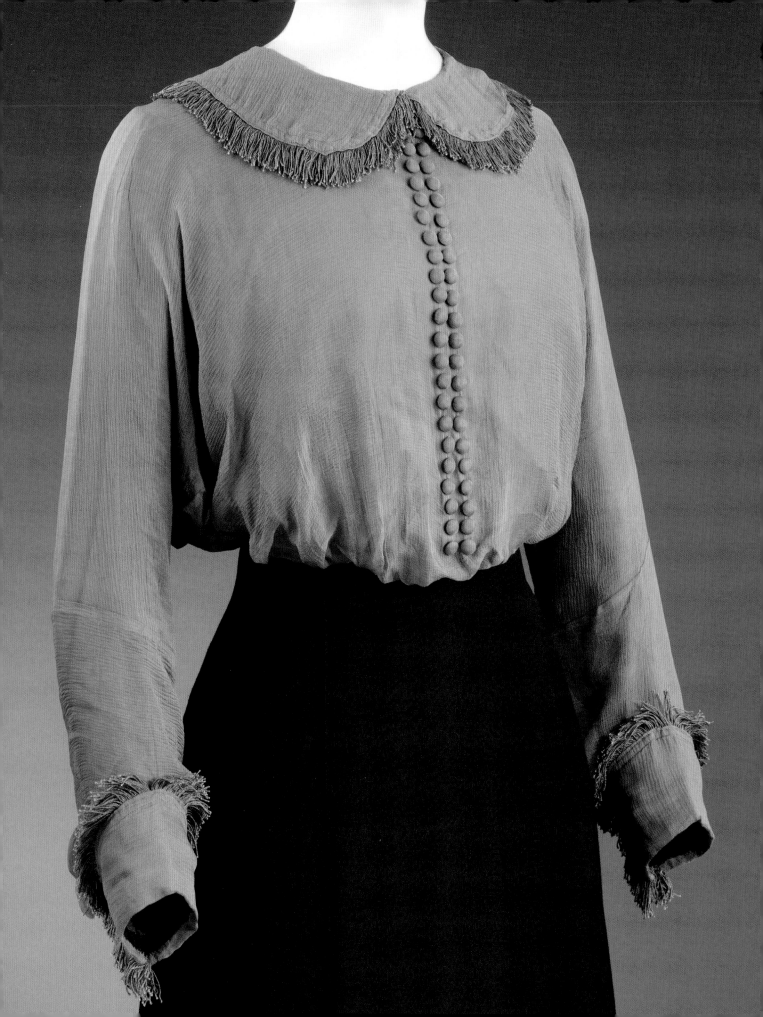

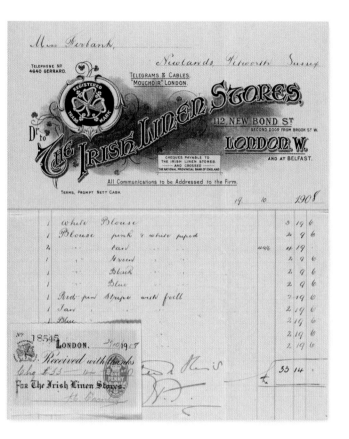

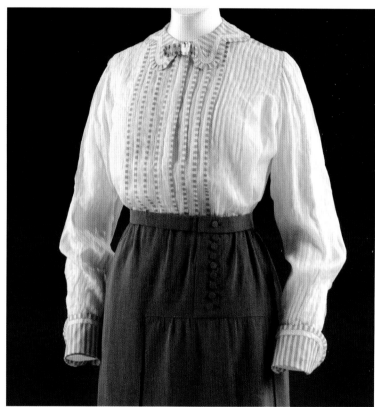

which they built their reputation. These are a silk velvet dinner dress [**47**] and a very fine black cashmere afternoon dress with a wired 'Tudor'-style collar and a bold purple cummerbund [**36**]. It dates from about 1913 and shows the Redfern response to the eclectic influences then affecting the direction of fashion. It is cut with batwing (known then as Magyar) sleeves and fastens asymmetrically at the front with press-studs hidden beneath non-functioning buttonholes with dropped Chinese-style buttons.

Redfern remained successful throughout and after the war, despite the subsequent changes in styles of dress and decline in demand for luxury clothes. In London they survived in various forms in collaboration with other companies until 1951.

BLOUSES

The blouse worn with a fine tailored costume developed as an important garment in the late nineteenth century, in parallel with the establishment of the tailor-made as a standard form of daywear. The earliest example in the Heather Firbank Collection [**38**] is high-necked and typically Edwardian, made of fine cotton, with intricate pin tucks and machine and chemical lace inserts,[10] worked over by hand with whitework embroidery – a style which fits with the earlier tailored costumes of around 1908. There is no maker's label on this blouse, but it has couture-quality hand-finishing and would undoubtedly have been labour-intensive to produce. Heather often bought many of her blouses in multiple colours in the same style from the Irish Linen Stores at 112 New Bond Street, which traded there from 1900

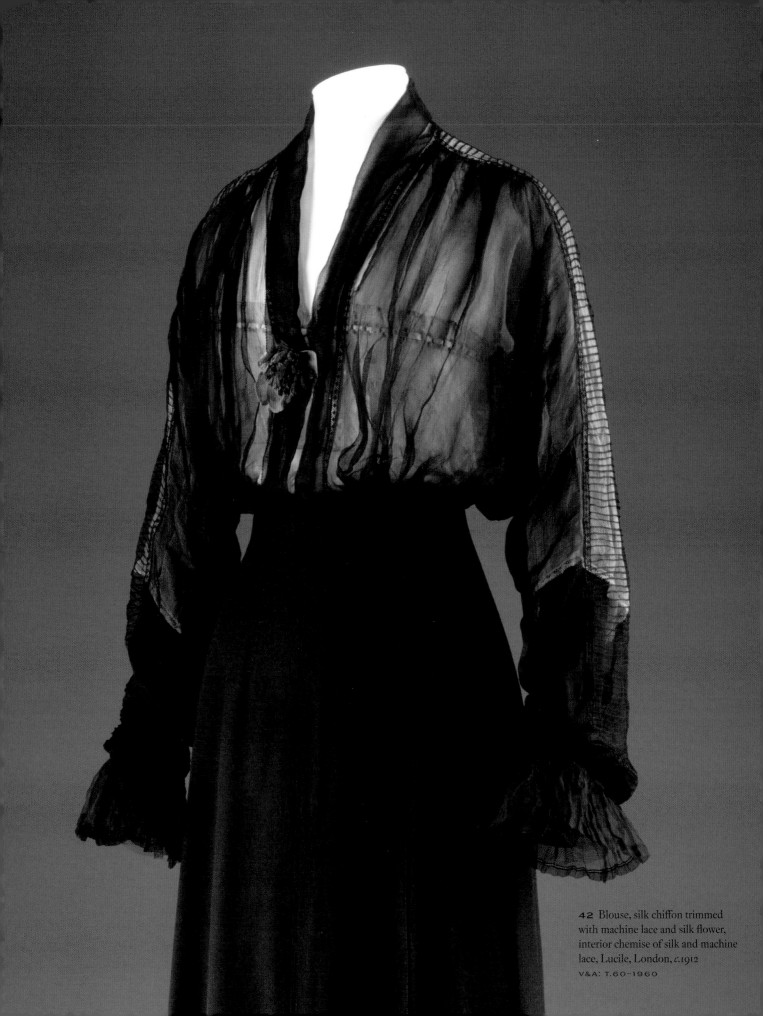

42 Blouse, silk chiffon trimmed
with machine lace and silk flower,
interior chemise of silk and machine
lace, Lucile, London, *c.*1912
V&A: T.60–1960

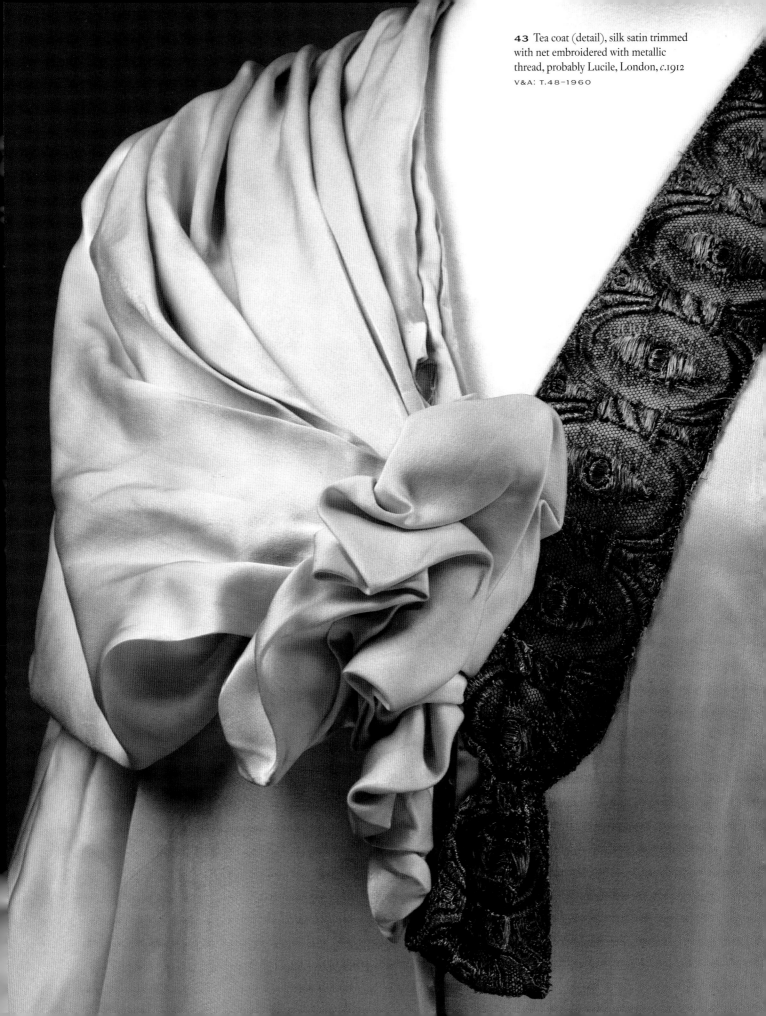

43 Tea coat (detail), silk satin trimmed
with net embroidered with metallic
thread, probably Lucile, London, *c.*1912
V&A: T.48–1960

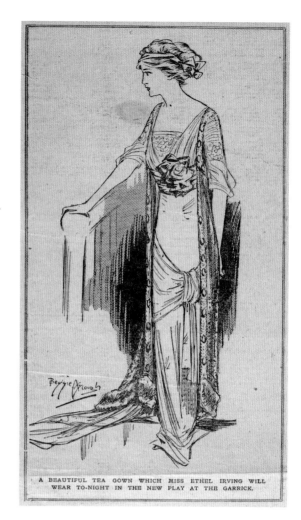

A BEAUTIFUL TEA GOWN WHICH MISS ETHEL IRVING WILL WEAR TO-NIGHT IN THE NEW PLAY AT THE GARRICK.

to 1925. A bill from the store dated 1908 describes a style in 'pin stripes with a frill', which corresponds very closely with surviving examples with stripes of green, black or red on a white ground with a modern flat collar and ruffles at the closing edges [**40, 41**]. A later development of the blouse as a garment in its own right is seen in Heather's silk examples from about 1912. Made by Lucile and by Mascotte, these were intended to be seen on informal occasions in the home, rather than to be hidden under a tailored jacket worn for daytime visiting or shopping [**42**]. The Mascotte example has a curved, flat collar of the sort that became known as the 'Peter Pan collar' after J.M. Barrie's character (*Peter Pan* was first performed in 1904 and was published as a novel in 1911) [**39**].

TEA GOWNS

On a day without formal engagements, Heather may have stayed in her day dress or tailor-made until the late afternoon, when she would have worn a tea gown before changing again for dinner. (Unfortunately, none of Heather's tea gowns survive in museum collections.) The tea gown was a highly specific and luxurious garment worn in the late afternoon or early evening when at home or staying at a country house [**44**]. It was considered a necessity for wealthy women from the late nineteenth to the early twentieth century. Less structured than dresses worn in public, it could be put on over a loosened corset and often had no internal stiffening. However, it was still a highly decorative garment, full-length and usually trimmed with a combination of lace, silk chiffon, beading, fur and faux flowers, and often a train. In 1901, *Lady's Realm* magazine described how women wore them: 'at five o'clock they will don the picturesque tea gown and adopt an air of drooping languor which savours of mystery, while striking an Oriental note of passion and colour.'[11]

Although the tea gown is often seen as the epitome of Edwardian frivolity and luxury, Heather's cuttings from fashion magazines show that this garment lived on well into the war years. One example in the *Daily*

Mail of 1915 depicts two tea gowns alongside an article entitled 'Good Temper Homes: How War Has Cured the Complaining Habit'. Shorter in length, in keeping with changing wartime fashions, it remained a luxurious item despite the austere climate, with trimmings including gold embroidery, gold tissue, purple chiffon, silver lace and chinchilla fur.

AFTERNOON DRESS

If a formal afternoon engagement had been arranged, another change was required – out of one's day dress or tailor-made and into a more elaborate gown known as an afternoon dress. This could come in many difficult-to-define forms. A cutting from Heather's collection showing labelled photographs of women wearing dresses for different times of day suggests that even at the time guidelines were necessary [**45**]. Dresses for afternoon occasions such as visits to garden parties were full-length, had more intricate trimmings than day dresses and often had a slight train. Unlike evening dress, however, they had

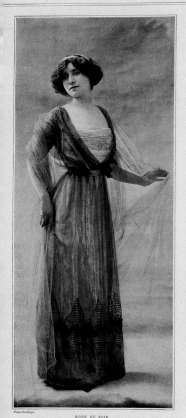
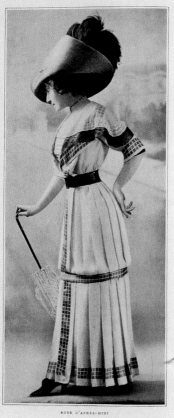
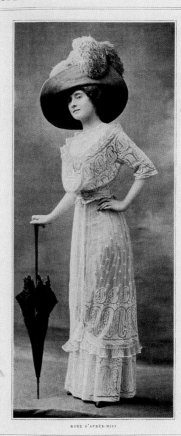
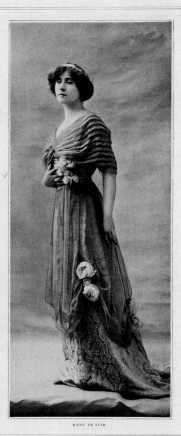

ROBE DU SOIR   ROBE D'APRÈS-MIDI   ROBE D'APRÈS-MIDI   ROBE DU SOIR

Mlle RENÉE DESPREZ

TOILETTES DE DOUCET

full- or half-length sleeves and high necks, and unlike tea gowns they were highly structured garments. An afternoon dress would have been worn with a wide, elaborate hat and a parasol in the summer. For social highlights such as the racing at Ascot or polo at the Ranelagh Club in south-west London, the trimmings could be almost as extravagant as on evening wear.

Heather's pale lilac silk dress, made by Mrs Pickett of the prestigious Savile Row, is a typical example of an afternoon dress [46]. Its high neckline and elbow-length sleeves mark it out as appropriate for this time of day. The silk satin of the main garment is overlaid with a grey/lilac silk chiffon. A border of machine-embroidered net and four decorative buttons on the chest are caught between these layers, casting the whole ensemble in a soft focus evocative of the 'endless summer' of the Edwardian era. The chiffon overlayer is parted at the front and gathered at two points at the rear, with the whole lot drawn into a decorative buckle at the back. The buckle is inspired by 1780s fashions, which were popular at the time.

EVENING DRESS

The type of dress worn in the evening had to be selected with great care – as Margot Asquith had found to her cost. Dinner dresses had low-cut necklines (though not off the shoulders) and often mid-length sleeves. Heather's black silk velvet dress, with its low, square neck and elbow-length sleeves, is an appropriate style for wearing to a dinner [47]. The thick, heavy silk velvet and its voluminous layered skirt and long train suggest it was for a formal winter dinner party. The dress, which was bought from Redfern, has a seventeenth-century-style trimming of a deep lace collar and cuffs of chemical lace. Diamanté details at the neckline and buttons defining the waist add a theatrical element.

The most formal evening dresses were those worn for balls. Ball gowns were full-length with a slight train, but, paradoxically, were the most revealing, with off-the-shoulder necklines and almost no sleeves, just wisps of chiffon over each shoulder. Heather's fantastical gold ball gown of around 1909

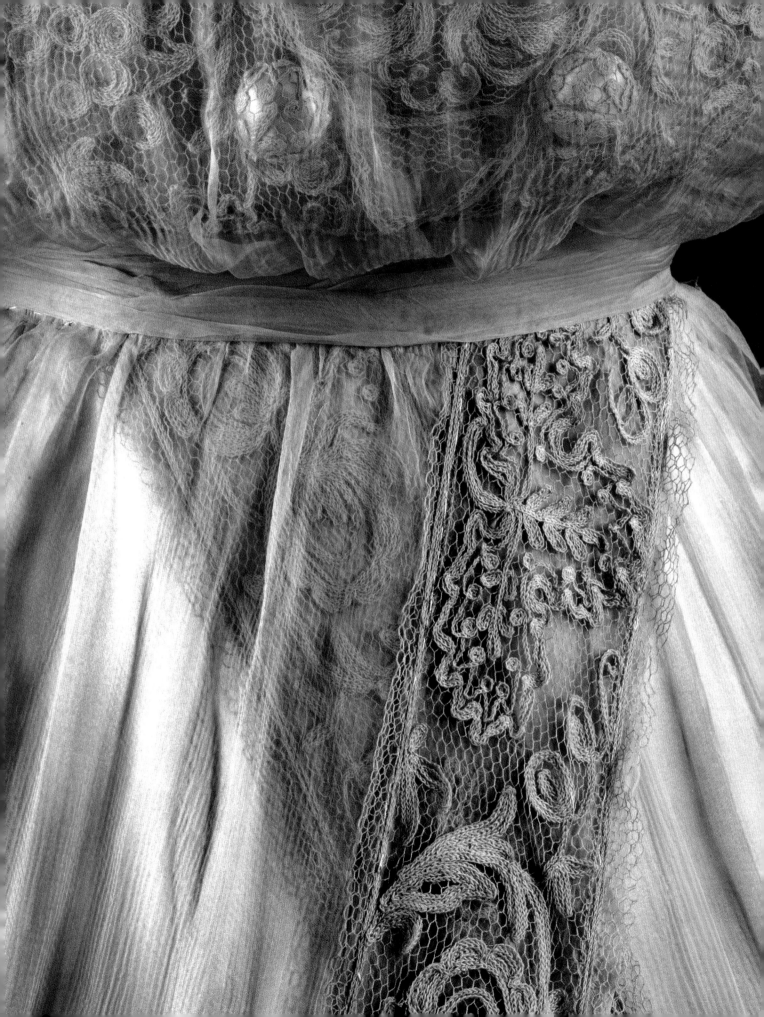

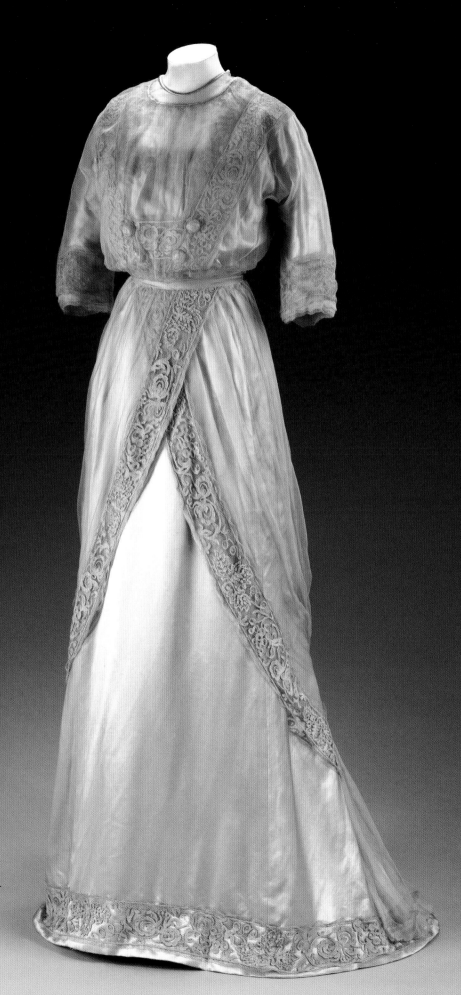

46 Afternoon dress, silk satin and silk chiffon, trimmed with machine-embroidered net, Pickett, London, c.1909
V&A: T.33-1960

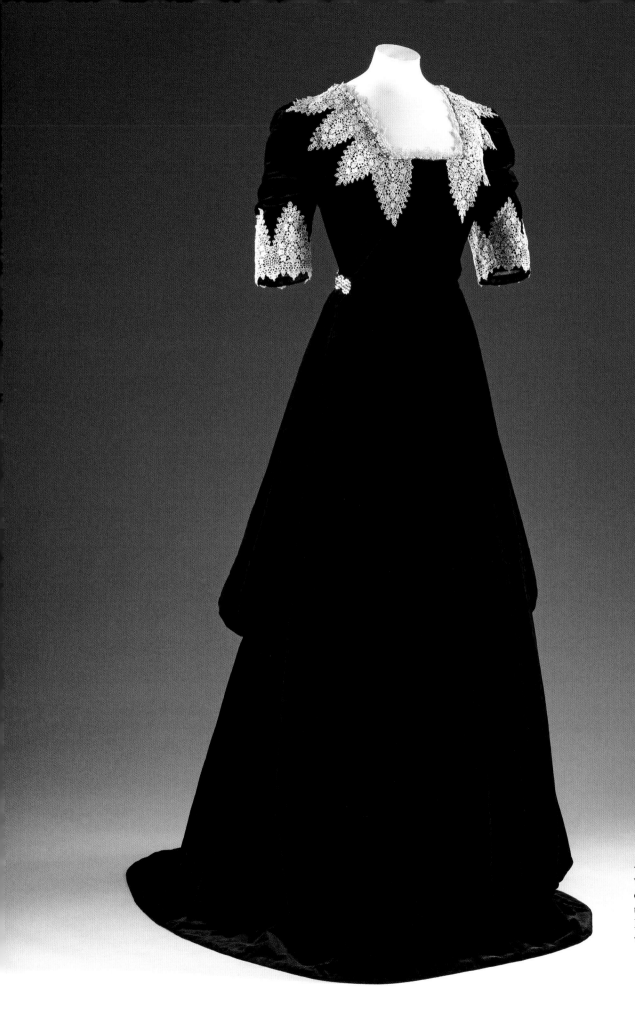

47 Dinner dress, silk velvet with chemical-lace collar and diamanté trimmings, Redfern, London, *c.*1909

V&A: T.29–1960

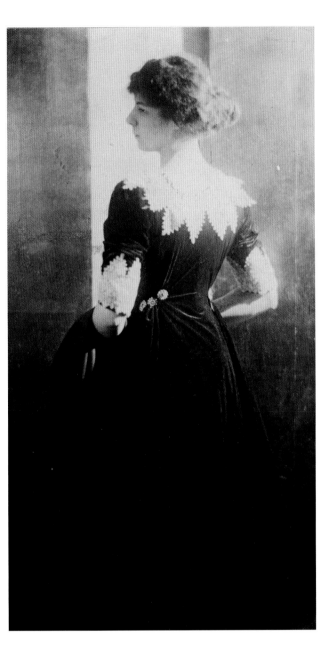

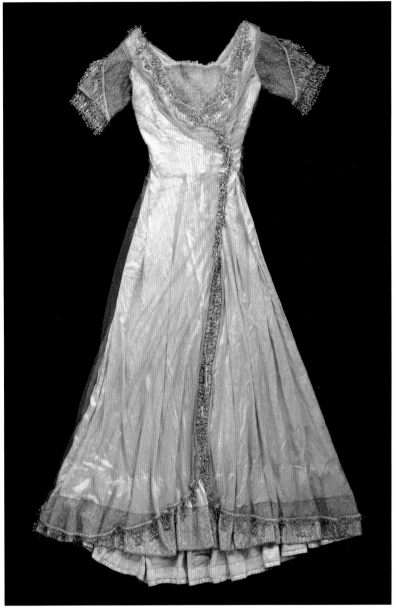

is typical of the light-coloured, delicately feminine ball dresses worn by young debutantes [**49**, and see **22**, **126**]. Decorated with a fine overlayer of silk net dotted with amber glass spots and silver beading around the décolletage and sleeves, it has no maker's label, although it would have undoubtedly been made bespoke for Heather by a court dressmaker, possibly Reville & Rossiter or Lucile. In keeping with changing fashions, the waist is just above natural height and the line is straight rather than in an 'S' bend.

Several of Heather's accessories from this period also survive, providing a rare opportunity to assemble

48 Heather Firbank wearing dress in plate 47, photographed by Baron Adolph de Meyer, *c*.1909
V&A: 8B-1974

49 Ball dress, silk satin with beaded net, trimmed with silver gilt machine lace and bugle beads, British, *c*.1909
V&A: T.47-1960

a full evening ensemble from items which might have been worn together. Her gold ball gown would have been worn with her white kid leather gloves extending well above the elbows [**146**], her gold court shoes [**51**] and possibly even her headdress imitating a garland of leaves [**50**].

50 Evening headdress, gilt wire with silk laurel leaves, British, 1908–10
V&A: T.132–1960

51 Pair of shoes, leather with diamanté decoration, Charles Lee, London, 1908–10
V&A: T.146&A–1960

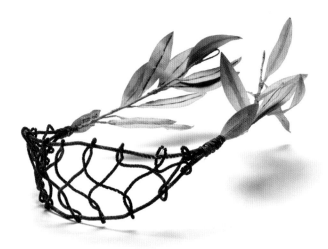

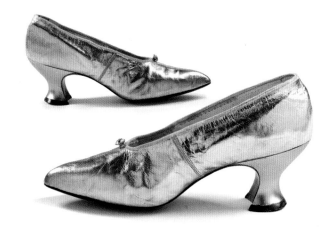

JEWELLERY

Apart from her wedding dress, one of the few items a young woman who moved in court and upper-class circles was not expected to buy from her allowance was jewellery. These key sartorial items were family heirlooms and carried a great weight of family history: the older the jewellery, the more status accrued to the wearer. Jewellery represented a woman's marital position and was the highest-status item in any Edwardian society woman's wardrobe. Family jewels were most often in the form of a matching set known as a parure, which contained a tiara, a large formal necklace, a hair ornament and elaborate matching earrings and bracelets, all worn for the grandest of social events and made in modular pieces so they could be altered in style from one generation to another. The parure was passed down to the eldest son and heir and worn by his wife. Thus women rarely if ever bought their own jewels. In a scene set in 1906 in Vita Sackville-West's novel *The Edwardians*, the Duchess of Chevron reflects on relinquishing her jewels:

She had recently had the family jewels reset by Cartier, preferring the fashions of the day to the heavy gold settings of Victoria's time. The top of the dressing-table was of looking-glass, so that the gems were duplicated; rubies to-night, she thought idly, picking up a brooch and setting it down again; last night she had worn the emeralds, and her depression returned as she reflected that some day she would have to give up the jewels to Sebastian's wife.[12]

Debutantes, no matter their families' wealth, wore delicate, light jewellery, considered suitable for young women, commonly strands of small pearls; expensive stones and diamonds were not seen as appropriate for young women. Heather owned an interlocking double-heart brooch which she wore in several of her debutante photos and this seems to have been a favourite piece [see 1]. A photograph of Heather's mother, taken by the Lafayette Studio in 1899, before her husband was knighted in 1902, shows her in court presentation dress, wearing an elaborate collection of pearl jewellery consisting of two necklaces, a cross-shaped choker, drop earrings and a matching jewelled hair comb. This may have been the family parure, although it is unlikely as it does not seem to be a set [see 8]. Heather, who remained unmarried, was almost certainly denied the opportunity to wear a striking and complete parure, although pieces of less valuable jewellery would have been gifted to her by her family.

HAIR AND HATS

Some of the most revealing insights into the creation and maintenance of a fashionable image are to be found among the more mundane purchases documented by Heather's bills. The shop Floris, described as 'Perfumer, Comb and Brush Maker' of Jermyn Street, provided Heather not only with scent but also with many different types of hair combs, in tortoiseshell and imitation jade. Her lady's maid, Adelaide Hallett, was very likely to have been a competent hairdresser, but Heather also went to the hairdresser Albert Minty, who was based at the Hyde Park Hotel. A bill from 15 January 1909 details four packets of hairpins at sixpence each and four bottles of shampoo powder at two shillings and sixpence each. A separate charge for 'combing made in puffs' demonstrates an effective method for building up hair into the required styles of the time. Cecil Beaton's description of his mother's hairdressing conveys something of the efforts that went into the elaborate coiffures of an Edwardian lady:

Since she had no personal maid, my mother was usually obliged to dress her own hair. It was worn wide at the sides, stuffed out with pads and garnished with amber tortoiseshell, or imitation diamond combs. On black Mondays, after a long solitary session with her arms upraised, putting the waves and curls into place, the effect might still not please her.

On special occasions a man with a moustache and sepia wavy hair parted in the centre would come to the house with a brown leather bag. He was shown to my mother's bedroom, where, armed with the spirit lamp or stove, he heated his tongs over a blue flame. I can still in memory conjure up the exciting scent of methylated spirit and singed hair.[13]

An uncovered head outdoors and in public remained taboo for the first half of the twentieth century, and in the early twentieth century hats became ever wider to accommodate the extravagant hairstyles. While much of the earlier Edwardian dress in Heather's wardrobe is understated and pared back, like many women of the period she indulged in flamboyant and theatrical millinery [55]. Many of Heather's hats – 16 of the 38 in the collection – were purchased from Woolland Brothers, the high-end department store in Knightsbridge, and had most likely been bought by them from Parisian milliners. Although Heather did not shop in Paris, many of the dressmakers she patronized made a feature of their French influence, copying French models and even adopting French names. One hat in the collection shows a French label giving the '*prix*' or price in French francs hidden under the Woollands' label [52]. In another example, inside the crown of a Woollands' labelled hat an additional label for the Paris couturière Suzanne Talbot reveals its original source.

Elaborate millinery reached a pinnacle in the Edwardian period, with hats supporting ever more fantastic trimmings. Among Heather's purchases were hats trimmed with silk flowers, fur, feathers and

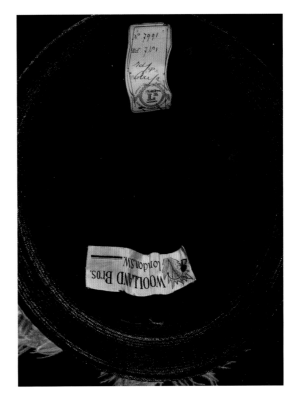

53 *below* Picture hat, plaited black straw, trimmed with cotton wisteria, Henry, London, 1908–10
V&A: T.105–1960

54 *right* Hat, covered with silk plush, trimmed with fur and feathers, Woolland Brothers, London, c.1910
V&A: T.106–1960

55 *left* Hat, covered with silk satin, trimmed with bird wing, Woolland Brothers, London, c.1910
V&A: T.104–1960

56 *below* 'Blériot' hat, straw faced with velvet, trimmed with feathers, René, Brighton, c.1911
V&A: T.115–1960

57 *bottom* Hat, plaited straw, trimmed with velvet flowers, Lucile, London, c.1920
V&A: T.113–1960

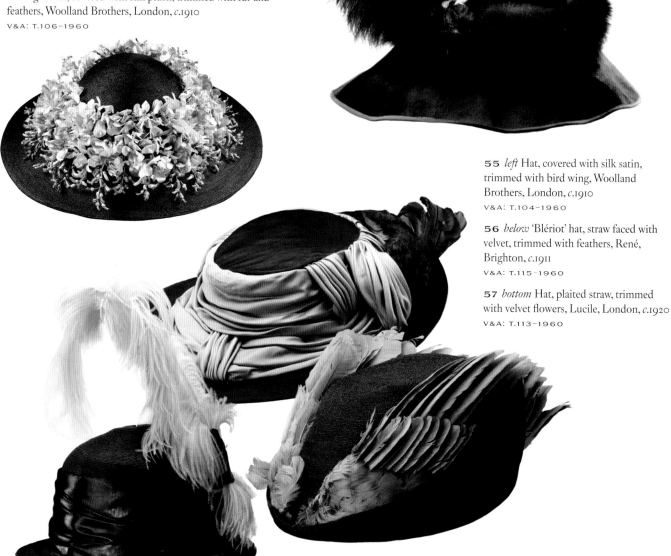

58 *above* Cloche hat with 'willow' plume, plaited straw and waxed ribbon, trimmed with ostrich and egret feathers, Woolland Brothers, London, c.1913
V&A: T.109–1960

59 *below* Picture hat, covered with silk, trimmed with silk flowers and ribbon, Woolland Brothers, London, c.1910
V&A: T.108–1960

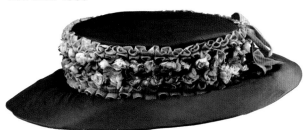

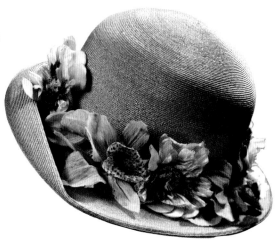

60 *top* Hat, plaited straw, trimmed with silk ribbon, Woolland Brothers, London, *c*.1910
V&A: T.120–1960

61 *below* Hat (detail) showing silk rose, British, *c*.1910
V&A: T.114–1960

62 *bottom* Picture hat, plaited straw, trimmed with ostrich feathers and dried barley, Suzanne Talbot, Paris, *c*.1910
V&A: T.235–1960

63 Cutting from *The Onlooker*, 31 October 1908
V&A: HEATHER FIRBANK ARCHIVE

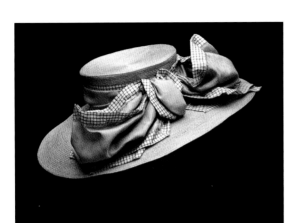

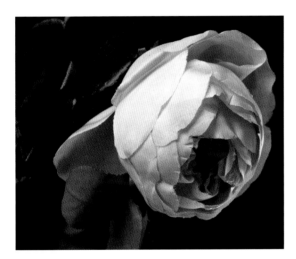

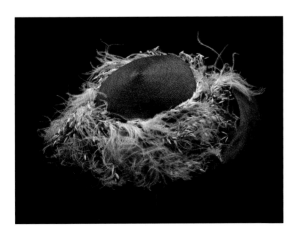

in some cases whole birds of every colour and style. Her black plaited straw hat trimmed with velvet and mounted with a pair of composite turquoise blue wings has been padded inside to ensure that the enlarged crown stayed perched on Heather's head [56]. This type of hat was known as a 'Blériot', after the first cross-Channel flight by French aviator Louis Blériot in 1909. The hat, which is labelled 'René of Brighton', would have been appropriate for wearing with a tailor-made costume in spring or autumn. More appropriate for summer, and reminiscent of Edwardian summer garden parties, is Heather's large straw hat trimmed with a profusion of silk wisteria flowers, from the milliner Henry, on Dover Street in Mayfair [53]. These hats would have been secured to her hair using decorative pins, which have left holes in the undersides and linings. The weight and

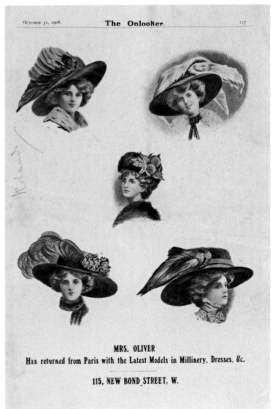

OCTOBER 31, 1908. **The Onlooker.** 117

MRS. OLIVER
Has returned from Paris with the Latest Models in Millinery, Dresses, &c.

115, NEW BOND STREET, W.

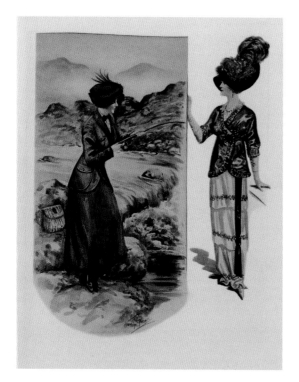

breadth of the hats must have caused considerable discomfort to the wearer, especially if it was windy, and women often pulled pale chiffon scarves over the top and fastened them under their chin to keep the hats in place.

Although women's hats had grown in size gradually since the start of the century, the vogue for exaggerated height, width and trimmings was cemented by the collaboration between high fashion and the popular theatre with the 1907 production of *The Merry Widow*, starring new actress and beauty Lily Elsie. Elsie's costumes for the production, designed by Lucile, included delicate silk and chiffon dresses and wide, deep hats piled with silks, feathers and flowers. The production was an international success and made a star of Elsie, while the 'Merry Widow' hat became a staple of the fashionable lady's wardrobe. Hats such as these, also known as 'picture hats' since they took their inspiration from eighteenth-century paintings by the likes of Gainsborough and

Reynolds, reached their most elaborate and extreme around 1912. From this point, they began to get smaller, moving towards the low-brimmed cloche-style hats of the 1920s. Heather's later millinery followed this trend, becoming more understated.

THE END OF THE SEASON: COUNTRY HOUSE VISITING

As Marcel Boulestin later recalled, once August arrived the London season ended:

The West End would be empty, the houses had closed; no more receptions, no more balls, for in a few days Goodwood races would be taking place, after which one could no longer be seen in London. Some left for their country houses, others for the beaches of Brittany and Normandy, before going north on the 12th of August to kill a few birds in Scotland or Yorkshire. The Season was over.[14]

August, September and October were usually spent in Scotland for a series of shooting, fishing and hunting trips and related hunt balls, with Christmas in London and then spring in Biarritz, Deauville or the South of France. Wealthy and well-connected families had homes in most of these places. Consequently, Boulestin noted, the aristocracy and upper middle classes only lived in their large London houses 'for about three months of the year'. Members of this circle would entertain each other on their country estates over long weekends – with dinners, parties, fancy-dress balls, hunting, shooting, sightseeing, church attendance, amateur theatricals, garden parties and so on. He added that 'a great number of indispensable domestic servants were required' because these country houses 'were not yet equipped with what are known as "modern conveniences"'.[15]

Country house visiting was a regular activity for wealthy young unmarried women and Heather would have enjoyed many such visits. As usual, it was vital to have exactly the right clothes for all occasions and to know when, where and how to wear them. Cynthia

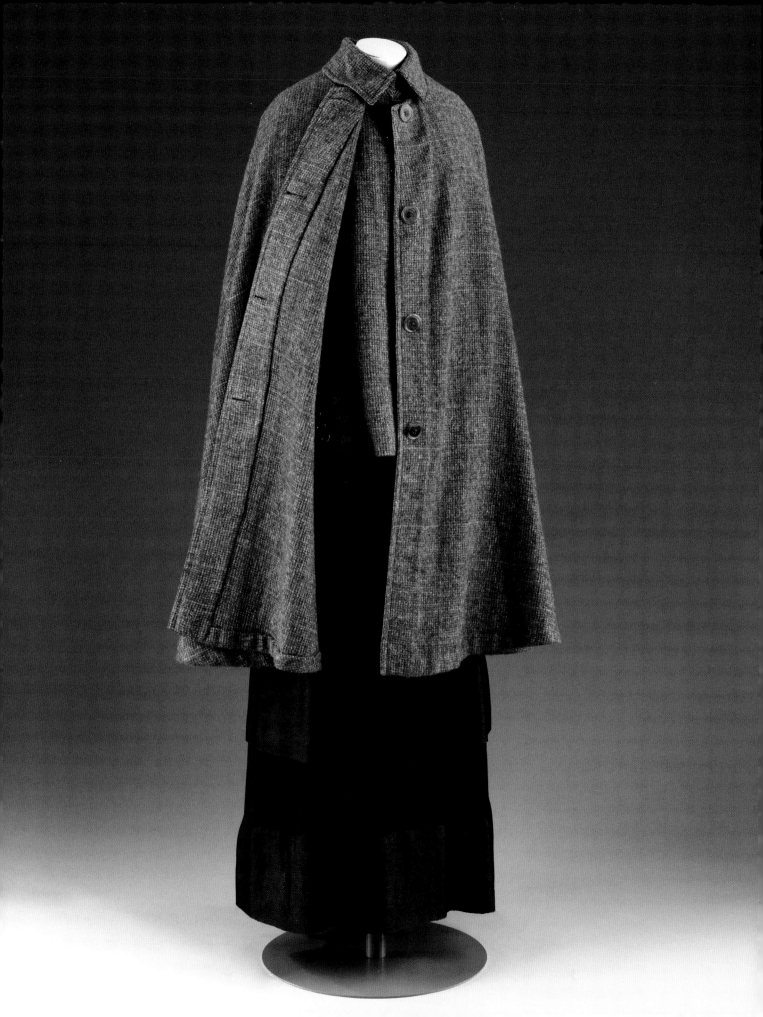

66 *The Bystander Hunting Supplement*, 14 October 1908
V&A: HEATHER FIRBANK ARCHIVE

67 Riding habit, tailored wool jacket, skirt and breeches,
cotton cravat and riding crop, Redfern, London, 1911, worn
by Mrs James Fraser
V&A: T.333A-D-1982

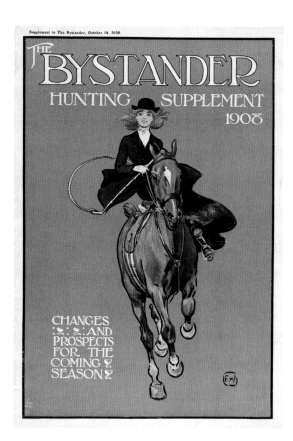

Asquith, Heather's contemporary, commented on the
pressures of dressing for a country house weekend:

*A large fraction of our time was spent in changing
our clothes, particularly in the winter, when you
came down to breakfast ready for church in your 'best
dress', made probably of velvet if you could afford it,
of velveteen if you couldn't. After church you went
into tweeds. You always changed again before tea,
into a 'tea gown' if you possessed that special creation;
the less affluent wore a summer day frock. However
small your dress allowance, a different dinner dress
for each night was considered necessary.*

Heather's clothing met all of these requirements in
the finest style, and only velvet, made of fine silk, and
not velveteen, an alternative made with cotton, would
have been found in her wardrobe.

In her account of her debutante years, Asquith
listed the sartorial requirements for just one weekend
in the country as follows:

*Your Sunday best, two tweed coats and skirts with
appropriate shirts, three evening frocks. Three garments suitable for tea, your 'best hat' – probably a
vast affair loaded with feathers, flowers, fruit or
corn – a variety of country hats and caps, as likely as
not a riding habit and billycock hat, rows of indoor
and outdoor shoes, boots and gaiters, numberless
accessories in the way of petticoats, shawls, scarves,
ornamental combs and wreaths and a large bag in
which to carry your embroidery about the house.*

She noted that taking all these garments with their
matching accessories necessitated 'at least one huge
domed trunk ... an immense hat-box and a heavy
dressing-case'.[16]

We know from surviving letters and papers that
Heather Firbank's country weekends included a
stay at Pitshill House, the home of Colonel William
Mitford, his wife, Cicely, and family, in Tillington,
near Petworth, around 1910, and that the expensive
luggage she required for such visits was purchased in
Bond Street and stamped with her initials.[17]

A SPORTING WARDROBE

The need for outdoor clothing for women was well
established by the 1900s. It was in the mid-nineteenth
century, following the example of Queen Victoria
with her enthusiasm for Highland walks, that well-
to-do women began to take up walking, shooting and
golfing. As well as a fashionable city lifestyle, Heather
also enjoyed country pursuits, including golf, skiing
and ice-skating. Specific garments were required for
each of these activities, which Heather bought from
the very best suppliers. Women's sportswear of all
types, using fabrics such as jersey and tweed, in practical, easy-to-wear styles, informed the movement
towards greater comfort and simplicity that came to
define the post-war wardrobe. However, even by the
early twentieth century comfort remained less important than propriety, and restrictive fashionable dress
codes still ruled.

A tailored riding habit was a basic component of
any aristocratic woman's wardrobe [**67**], and although
Heather's no longer survives, we have numerous
photographs of her horses and copies of her riding magazines. Furthermore, Heather's great-niece
Johanna Firbank recalls that Heather was a good
horsewoman and enjoyed hunting; the family still
have her extravagant jewelled horse whip. Costumes

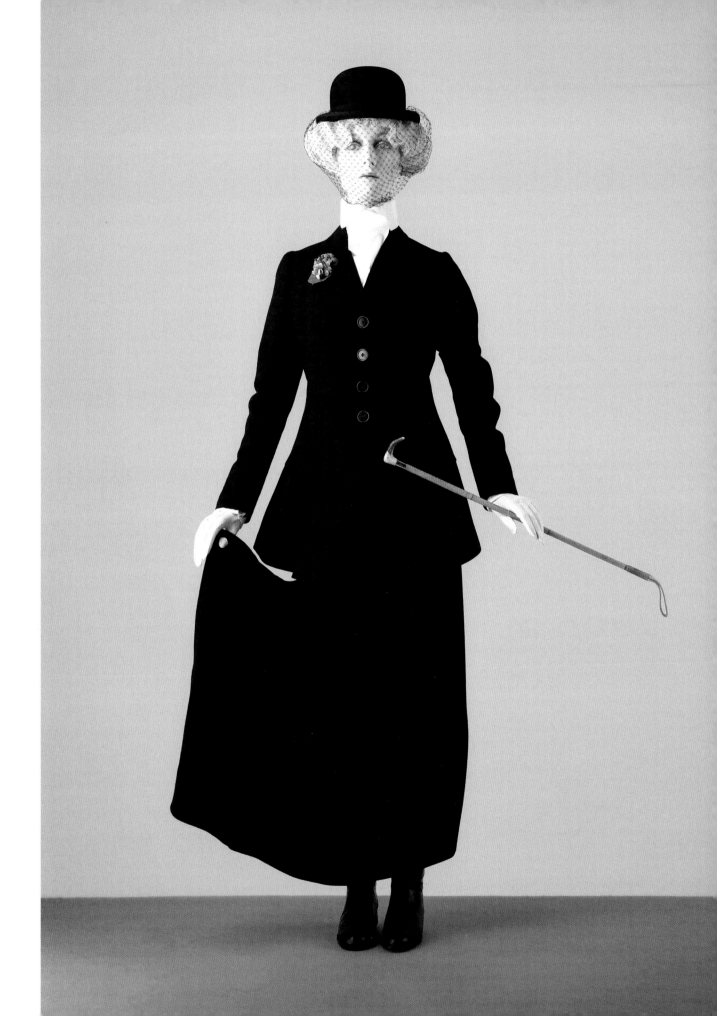

68 'Pursuing the Partridges', cutting from *Tatler*,
11 October 1911
V&A: HEATHER FIRBANK ARCHIVE

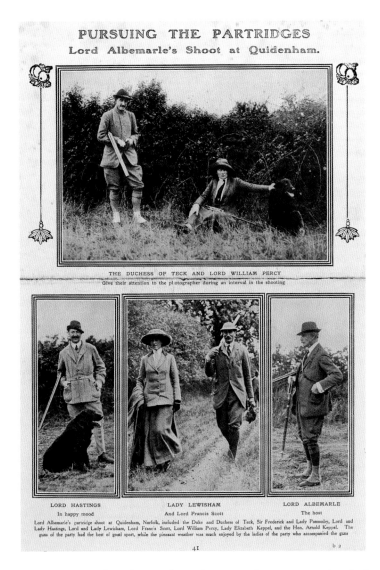

PURSUING THE PARTRIDGES
Lord Albemarle's Shoot at Quidenham.

THE DUCHESS OF TECK AND LORD WILLIAM PERCY
Give their attention to the photographer during an interval in the shooting

LORD HASTINGS
In happy mood

LADY LEWISHAM
And Lord Francis Scott

LORD ALBEMARLE
The host

Lord Albemarle's partridge shoot at Quidenham, Norfolk, included the Duke and Duchess of Teck, Sir Frederick and Lady Ponsonby, Lord and Lady Hastings, Lord and Lady Lewisham, Lord Francis Scott, Lord William Percy, Lady Elizabeth Keppel, and the Hon. Arnold Keppel. The guns of the party had the best of good sport, while the pleasant weather was much enjoyed by the ladies of the party who accompanied the guns

41

women's tailored garments were an industry in their own right and Heather would have visited one of the many supplying sportswear, most likely Redfern or Frederick Bosworth, from whom she purchased her other tailored costumes.

For sporting activities during a country house weekend tweeds were another important staple [**68**]. Heather had good-quality examples made by specialist suppliers such as Scott Adie, royal cloak maker and owner of the Royal Scotch Warehouse.[18] Worn for game shooting – women would not usually have taken part themselves, but would have walked alongside the shooters and beaters, stopping to enjoy an elaborate outdoor luncheon – Heather's Scott Adie cloak is made of the finest 'homespun' (coarse and hand-woven) tweed, with a delicate blue and orange line running through. There is a close-fitting inner waistcoat which buttons down the front and has large pockets, with the cloak of matching fabric attached at the back. The garment is heavy and hard-wearing but beautifully finished, with every care taken to match up the tweed design at the seams and hems [**65**]. The large silk label on the inside reads: 'Waterproof Cloak Maker to Her Majesty the Queen, The Princess of Wales and All the Foreign Courts'.

For golfing Heather owned a very fine tailored ensemble comprising jacket, skirt and tam-o'-shanter-style cap made of homespun black and brown Scottish tweed, dating from about 1908 – the only piece of her sportswear in the V&A collections [**69**].[19] Both the cap and jacket are lined with cream silk and labelled with the maker, 'Frederick Bosworth, Ladies Tailor and Court Dressmaker'. The attention to detail in Heather's golfing ensemble highlights the high quality of Bosworth's workmanship. Hand-stitched, tan-leather trimmings reinforce the areas of greatest wear at the cuffs, pockets and buttons; an extra band of fabric is used to weight the skirt at the hem to prevent it blowing up in high winds; the pockets at the front open in two ways; a hook and eye fastening at the back of the skirt enables the closing of a box pleat to take in fabric and make the skirt narrower if

for riding in the early twentieth century consisted of a tailored jacket, breeches, skirt and hat, often in the style of a smaller version of a man's top hat. Women would have ridden sidesaddle and the breeches of the riding habit would have been fashioned in black fabric so as to go unnoticed if the overskirt was caught by the wind (although skirts were constructed with straps to prevent this). Riding habits were the earliest garments to be made for women by a tailor, often their husband's or father's. However, by the 1900s

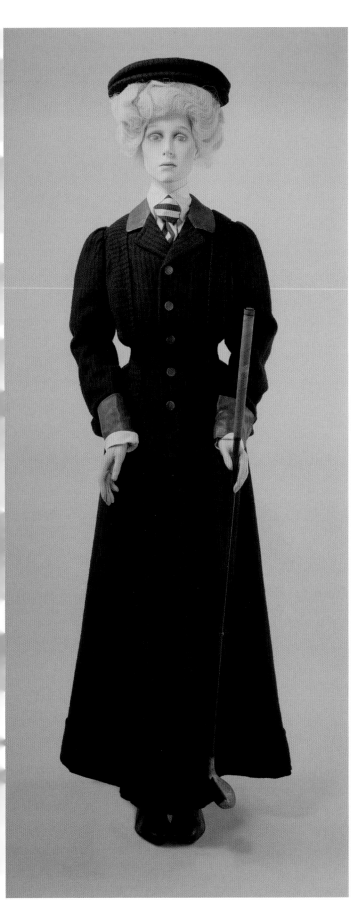

69 Golfing ensemble, tailored jacket, skirt and cap, 'homespun' tweed trimmed with leather, Frederick Bosworth, London, 1905–8
V&A: T.20A–D–1960

preferred; and the tweed design is expertly aligned at every seam. The length of the skirt, although shorter than in a city walking costume to allow greater movement and to ensure that the fabric did not soak up water, remained only inches above the floor, and the corseted waist and high-collared shirt were also maintained despite their obvious restrictions. Having the correct fabric for the costume was crucial, and in wearing thick Highland tweed Heather was extremely fashionable. In summer 1897 the fashion journal *Gentlewoman* identified the most famous of the Highland tweeds, Harris tweed, as the 'leading fabric for smart gowns, destined to exploit the charms of lovely women on the moors, by the sea or ... cycling'.[20] Importantly, as Janice Helland notes, these fabrics were not designed for the Scottish market but for the urban upper-middle-class lady and her 'country moments'. Promoted as exclusive and unique, they were made all the more appealing by their 'otherness'.[21]

The two pairs of Heather's skiing trousers now at the Gallery of Costume in Manchester are examples of rare early-twentieth-century women's bifurcated garments. Before the war trousers were worn by women, if at all, only for sporting activities such as skiing or cycling and were often concealed by an overskirt. In the years after the war, with the general relaxation of attitudes to women in trousers due to those worn for war work, knickerbocker-style garments for skiing, worn with belted tunics, became more commonplace.[22] Both pairs are made of thick woollen cloth and have a detachable lining, presumably for ease of washing. The crotch of the trousers is low, to allow for ease of movement, and one pair has knitted woollen stockings attached, making an all-in-one stocking and trouser. The trousers would have been worn with matching jackets which unfortunately were not kept. There are no maker's labels on the trousers, but their quality suggests that, like the golfing ensemble, they were made by a notable tailor.

Although no tennis dress of Heather's survives, a photograph in the collection shows her posing in

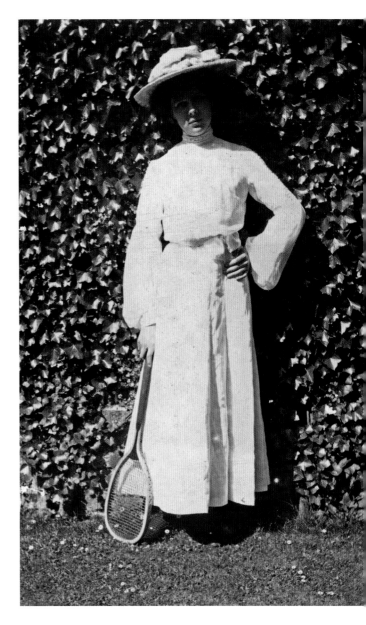

tennis clothes [**70**]. The high neck on the blouse, fabric gathered in at the waist and flared skirt date the picture to about 1905, when she would have been 17 years old. The clothing is light in colour for summer sports and, although still relatively restrictive for sportswear, the skirt is shorter, as she is a young woman. Heather maintained a keen interest in tennis and later in life donated land she owned as part of the St Julian's estate in Newport to build a tennis club, which is still known as the Firbank Dale Tennis Club.

By the 1900s motoring had become a sport among the upper classes. In an article in 1913 in *The Strand* reflecting on the rise of the motorcar, the author noted: 'The triumph of motoring began when a number of people discovered it was expensive. Then there was a rush of people who envy the distinction of incurring expense.'[23] Although there is no evidence that Heather ever drove a car herself – she would no doubt have been driven by a chauffeur – she had specific clothing for motoring, which included a long coat of twilled wool, purchased from Woolland Brothers, for warmth and protection in the early open-top vehicles, and a motoring cap of orange felt with a sporty-looking brim from Woodrow & Sons, which would have been held on by a light scarf tied beneath the chin.[24]

FASHIONABLE DISCOMFORTS

While the clothes of this period appear romantic and luxurious, they brought with them physical discomfort and even lack of hygiene. For an afternoon walk, even the shorter trains of daywear were lined at the hem with an interchangeable ruffle or 'balayeuse' which could be removed and washed. Nonetheless, as Cynthia Asquith recollected, 'Walking about the London streets trailing clouds of dust was horrid. I once found I had carried into the house a banana skin which had got caught up in the unstitched hem of my dress!'[25] Today we may admire the elegance and boldness of the decorated hats of the Edwardian era, but many women found them deeply inconvenient. Referring to the period between 1910 and 1912, when

hat veils were worn pulled down over the face outdoors, Asquith talked of them spoiling her 'vision with huge black spots like symptoms of liver trouble'. She complained that the 'vast hats ... were painfully skewered to our heads with the ornamental hat pin, greatly to the peril of other people's eyes'. She 'couldn't endure the high choking collars with boned supports that dug red dints in my neck', so 'wore low, square-necked blouses long before these became the fashion – a non-conformity for which I was severely criticized'. As elegant as Heather's country tweeds appear today, these were remembered with dread: 'Country tweeds were long and trammelling. Imagine the discomfort of a walk in the rain in a sodden skirt that wound its wetness round your legs and chapped your ankles.'[26]

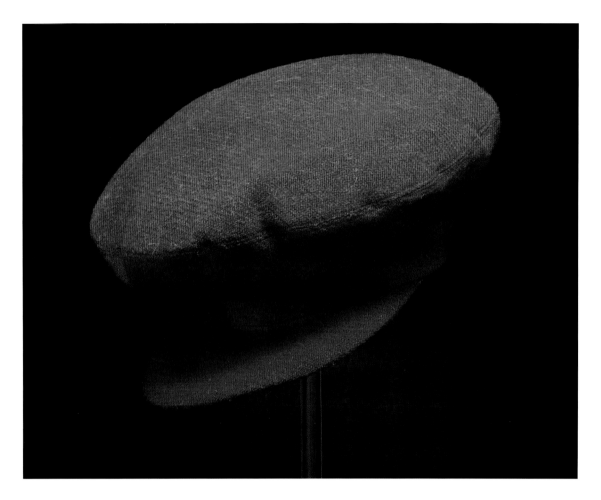

71 Motoring cap, wool tweed,
Woodrow, London, *c.*1910
V&A: T.130-1960

72 Interior detail of plate 71 showing padding, silk lining
and printed silk label

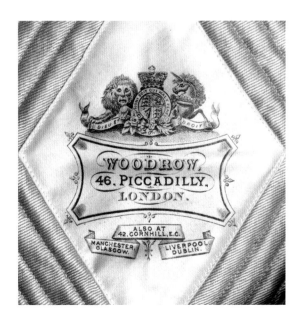

THE LADY'S MAID: MANAGING A WARDROBE

It was not enough simply to be able to buy the 'right' clothes for every occasion: an elegant woman also had to manage the garments she required. Cynthia Asquith remembered the help she needed, which was usually provided by a personal maid, 'perpetually making, mending, washing, darning and packing'. She also bemoaned the fact that women were 'humiliatingly dependent on help' because it was a 'physical impossibility to get in or out of [dresses] unassisted'.[27] Garments were closed at the back and were complicated by delicate layers of overlapping fabric, each one fastening with rows and rows of tiny hooks and eyes.

A description in Vita Sackville-West's novel *The Edwardians* gives an idea of the amount of work that went into getting dressed for a society ball:

[H]er mother would rise, and, standing in her chemise, would allow the maid to fit the long stays of pink coutil, heavily boned, around her hips and slender figure, fastening the busk down the front, after many adjustments; then the suspenders would

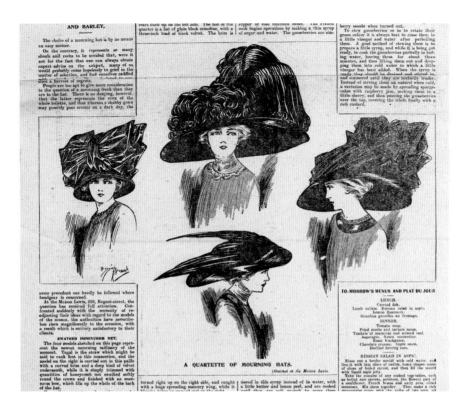

be clipped to the stockings; then the lacing would follow, beginning at the waist and travelling up and down, until the necessary proportions had been achieved. The silk laces and their tags would fly out, under the maid's deft fingers, with the flick of a skilled worker mending a net. Then the pads of pink satin would be brought, and fastened into place on the hips and under the arms, still further to accentuate the smallness of the waist. Then the drawers; and then the petticoat would be spread into a ring on the floor, and Lucy would step into it on her high-heeled shoes, allowing Button [the maid] to draw it up and tie the tapes ... She says 'Button, I am ready for my dress. Now be careful. Don't catch the hooks in my hair.' ... Button, gathering up the lovely mass of taffeta and tulle, held the bodice open while the Duchess flung off her wrap and dived gingerly into the billows of her dress ... the maid breathed a sigh of relief as she began doing up the innumerable hooks at the back.[28]

In 1910, when Heather was invited for a country weekend at Pitshill House, the home of Colonel William Mitford (an encounter that would later have a profound impact on her life), his wife, Cicely, instructed her 'to bring her maid' to help with her dressing and to ensure that her clothes were in proper order.[29]

In the 1911 census almost 1.3 million people were listed as being in service – even a modest middle-class household in the pre-war period would have had servants. Records show that Heather's lady's maid, Adelaide Hallett, came to work for the family at some time between 1901 and 1911 when in her early to mid-twenties. Before moving to the Firbank's Curzon Street home in Mayfair, where they lived from about 1909 to 1914, she was a boarder at the Young Women's Christian Association in Bournemouth together with 70 other young women. Her occupation, like that of many of the others, is listed as a dressmaker. Hallett was employed as lady's maid to Heather and her mother, and it would have been important for both women that she had dressmaking skills and a good knowledge of fashion.

Hallett would have been expected to tend to the Firbank ladies' toilette, washing and mending their clothes, styling their hair, helping them dress and even occasionally advising them on what to wear and buy. Hallett had a close and personal working relationship with Heather, and family letters reveal that she remained an important companion throughout her life. In the early 1920s Ronald suggested that Hallett chaperone Heather on a trip to Italy, when she could find nobody else (in fact, the trip did not go ahead). Later in life, when Heather was in less fortunate circumstances, it was Hallett who wrote on

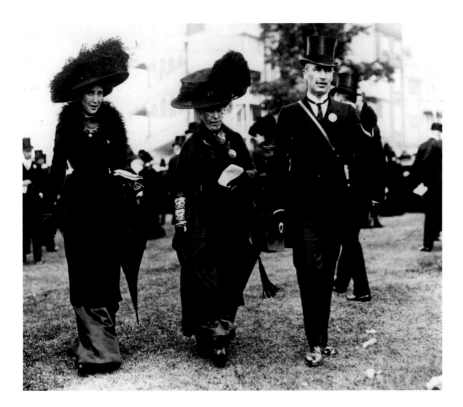

her behalf to Ronald to ask him to be sympathetic to his sister, and, as Heather had no surviving close relatives when she died, it was Hallett who inherited Heather's wardrobe and gave it to the V&A for a token sum of just £30.

MOURNING DRESS

Mourning dress was another major part of managing a wardrobe. After a family bereavement, the complexities of mourning-dress etiquette, including choice of fabric, jewellery and hats, were an additional strain to cope with. Women attached to court circles were also obliged to wear court mourning whenever it was decreed by the Lord Chamberlain.

Edward VII died on 6 May 1910, when Heather was 22. General court mourning, in which full black clothing was to be worn, was declared from 10 May until 18 June, followed by a further period of half-mourning, in which tones of black, grey, dull mauve and white would have been worn for a shorter period. Heather would have been obliged to keep this convention. Crinkled dull silk mourning crêpe, the fabric which had epitomized the respectable Victorian widow, was still worn on garments and hats [73], but was rivalled by black voile or georgette by the beginning of the twentieth century.[30] The *Evening Standard and St James's Gazette* warned on 10 May 1910 that:

the choice of mourning hats is by no means an easy matter. On the contrary, it represents so many shoals and rocks to be avoided that, were it not for the fact that one can always obtain expert advice on the subject, many of us would probably come hopelessly to grief in the matter of selection, and find ourselves saddled with ... a harvest of regrets.[31]

Marcel Boulestin remembered that 'it was strange to see the whole city in black, men, women and shops. Even those outside court circles, who were not compelled to wear full mourning, wore at least a black tie.'[32] On 14 May the *Illustrated London News* described the rush to the mourning suppliers, especially the smart department stores in London, which became 'literally besieged from morning to night'.[33] The season of 1910 became known as the 'Black Season'. At Ascot races that year, the colourful and flamboyant racegoing attire was replaced by mourning dress, with black ostrich feathers topping black hats and full-length black gowns to mark the death of the King [74].

The death of Edward VII less than 10 years after the death of Queen Victoria meant that mourning dress was especially visible and created a vogue for black clothing which ran parallel to the requirements for mourning. In the catalogues for Lucile's innovative mannequin parades of 1913, dresses clearly

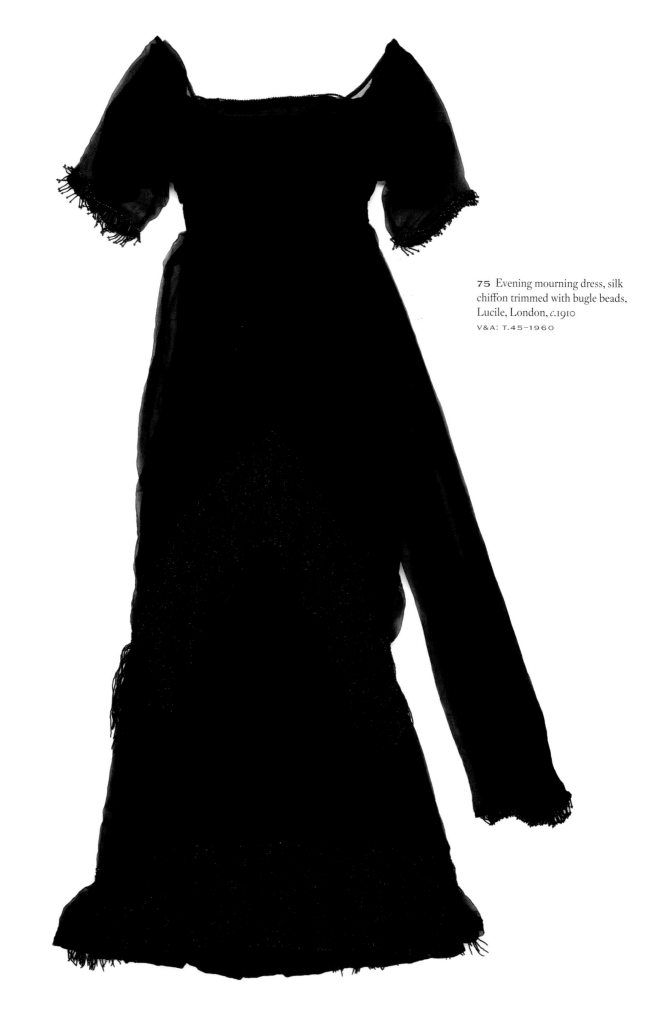

75 Evening mourning dress, silk
chiffon trimmed with bugle beads,
Lucile, London, *c.*1910
V&A: T.45–1960

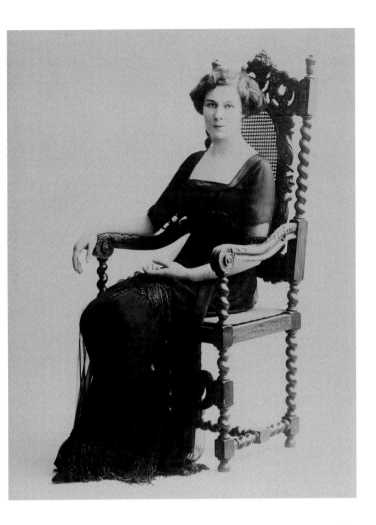

76 Heather Firbank wearing Lucile mourning dress in plate 75, photographed by Rita Martin, *c*.1910
V&A: HEATHER FIRBANK ARCHIVE

designed for mourning – given such names as 'In Sympathy' and '*Veuve Joyeuse*' (Merry Widow) – were offered alongside other designs in black such as '*Papita*', a black satin tango cloak, and 'Dear Lady Disdain', a black satin afternoon dress.[34]

HEATHER IN MOURNING

The Firbank family was frequently rocked by death and loss. Heather's adolescent wardrobe would have changed dramatically in 1904 when Joey, her oldest brother, died at Chislehurst, aged just 20, from a mystery illness and the family was plunged into mourning. Etiquette books at the time dictated that mourning dress should be worn for six months following the death of a sibling – full mourning for the first three months, followed by half-mourning for a further three.[35] These sombre colours reflected the emotional impact of the death on the young Heather, who was just 16. A letter from her brother Ronald consoles her and acknowledges what a shock this

must have been in her otherwise tranquil childhood. He wrote, 'There is bound to be ennui, when things become REAL.'[36] Heather and Ronald were very close and numerous letters between them survive. Although he spent most of his life abroad, he wrote to Heather, whom he called 'Baby', almost daily, remaining her confidant throughout his life.

In contrast to the light, feminine, optimistic evening gowns of her debutante year, some of the evening dresses and daywear that survive from two years later have a very different feel, again reflecting sad events in Heather's life. One such dress by Lucile, dated around 1910, is made of black silk chiffon with a black draped overskirt and a deep fringing of black beads on the sleeves, bodice and skirt [**75, 76**]. Different textures and trimmings are employed to create visual interest and a feeling of luxury in a garment which is exclusively black. The addition of sparkling jet beading suggests that this was worn for the slightly less austere half-mourning period rather than full mourning.[37] This could be an example of fashionable black clothing, but due to the sad events of this year is more likely to be mourning dress. For Heather this dress, and the many other black garments in the collection from this time, was probably worn to mourn her father, Thomas Firbank, who died suddenly, just four months after King Edward.

With the death of Thomas Firbank the family suffered not only emotional loss, but also the loss of the anchor of the family's wealth and status. All of the family's practical financial and property matters became the responsibility of Heather's oldest surviving brother, Ronald, who quickly realized that the Firbank fortune, although enough to maintain a comfortable upper-middle-class existence, was unstable and significantly smaller than they had believed.[38] He wrote cautionary letters to his mother and sister regarding their extravagant spending, which, as surviving dressmakers' bills reveal, seem to have made very little impact on the fashion-hungry Heather.

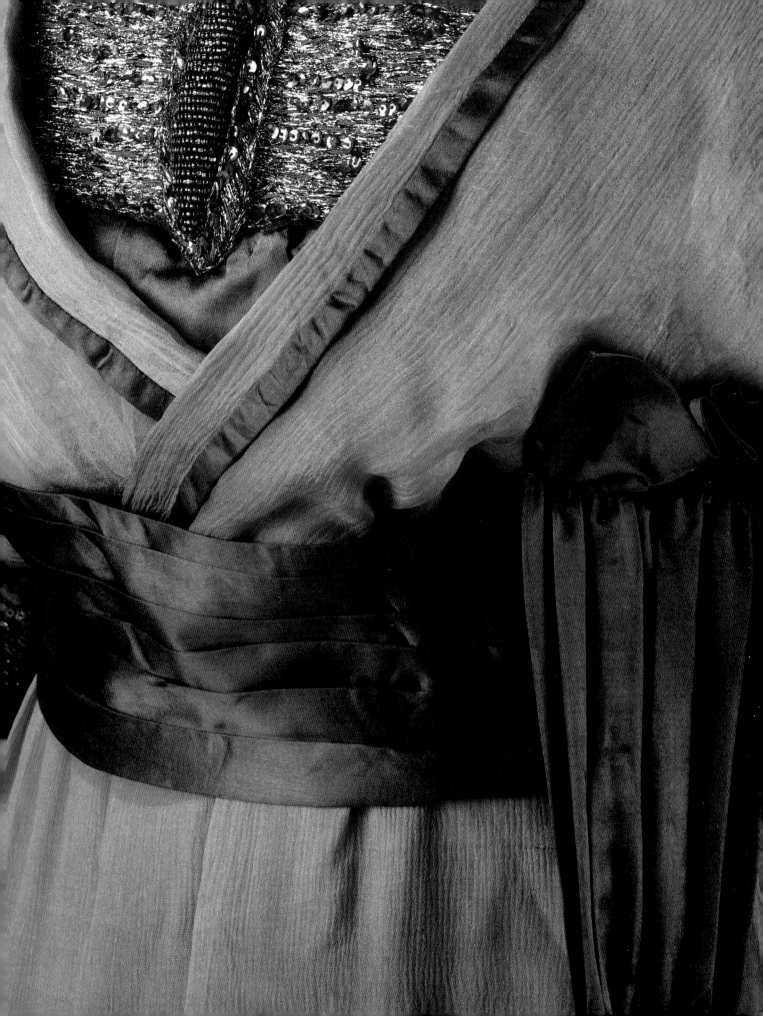

DISCRETIONS, INDISCRETIONS AND NONCONFORMITY IN SOCIETY LONDON
1910–14

On King Edward's death, his oldest surviving son, George, took the throne and he and his wife became King George V and Queen Mary. Officially the Edwardian era had come to a close, but in many ways its values and aesthetics continued until the outbreak of war in 1914. The new king and queen were more sober figureheads than Edward VII and his wife had been, providing a consistency and stoicism that would be highly valued in the war years to come. In the quarter-century that George V reigned, bohemianism, socialism, communism and fascism all grew in strength and changed the political and cultural landscape dramatically, but George held steadfastly to the values of the previous decade.

For the first years of the twentieth century, fashionable dress changed very little. Then, from about 1908, waistlines became higher, bosoms less pronounced and skirts narrower. As the new reign began, fashions started to change more rapidly, with new shapes emerging each season and new influences from the East arriving through the performances of Diaghilev's orientalist-inspired Ballets Russes, promoted most successfully by the work of French designer Paul Poiret.

Heather was 22 in 1910 and, still unmarried, was living with her mother at their relatively modest London residence in Curzon Street with a reduced staff of just four. When in the country, they stayed in an elegant, three-storey 1790s red-brick house in the village of Petworth. Here Heather socialized with the Hon. Margaret Blanche Wyndham, youngest daughter of Henry Wyndham, 2nd Lord Leconfield, whose great late-seventeenth-century home, Petworth House, overshadowed Pound Street, where the Firbanks' house stood. Heather maintained her interest in changing fashions and it was in her early twenties that her personal style was most adventurous and sophisticated.

LUCILE

Many of Heather's dresses from this time were bought from Lucile, the professional name of Lucy Sutherland, later Lady Duff-Gordon, who has become perhaps the most famous of the London court dressmakers and the designer who had the greatest influence on Heather's taste. This celebrity was partly thanks to her success in self-promotion and journalism, which culminated in a popular autobiography, *Discretions and Indiscretions* (1932). Lucile began her career by making dresses for friends and family to support herself and her daughter, having been divorced by her first husband, James Stuart Wallace. In 1894 she opened a shop in Old Burlington Street, moving to larger premises at 17 Hanover Square in 1897. Lucile developed a reputation for making distinctive tea gowns, building up a wealthy clientele which included notable names from the theatre. She claimed to have been responsible for introducing sensual, romantic lingerie and tea gowns, and sales techniques such as theatrical live fashion shows. She drew particular attention to her models, so that they became known in their own right. Giving her designs poetic names rather than numbers, she traded on the impression that they were created individually for clients as 'personality dresses', rather than being part of a pre-existing collection. Cecil Beaton described her designs in his memoirs:

77 Evening dress (detail of plate 83)

Lucile worked with soft materials, delicately sprin-
kling them with bead or sequin embroidery, with
cobweb lace insertions, true lovers' knots, and gar-
lands of minute roses. Her colour sense was so subtle
that the delicacy of detail could scarcely be seen at a
distance, though the effect she created was of an inde-
finable shimmer. Sometimes, however, she introduced
rainbow effects into a sash and would incorporate
quite vivid mauves and greens, perhaps even a touch
of shrimp-pink or orange. Occasionally, if she wanted
to be deliberately outrageous, she introduced a bit
of black chiffon or black velvet, and, just to give the
coup de grâce, outlined it with diamonds.[1]

Lucy married her second husband, Sir Cosmo Duff-
Gordon, in 1900, becoming Lady Duff-Gordon. She
is the best-known example of an aristocrat break-
ing through social barriers and earning a living in
'trade'. As she herself commented, once she started
to design and make couture clothes commercially,
she 'lost caste terribly'.[2] Advising wealthy American
women tourists on purchasing elegant clothing in
London, the writer and artist Blanche MacManus
confirmed that 'In London what are known as the
"West End" Court dressmakers are the aristocracy of
the profession, and not infrequently are members of
the aristocracy itself, pushed into business by necessity and often bringing with them their impecunious
lady friends as assistants.'[3]

    In 1904 the shop moved to a large Georgian man-
sion at 23 Hanover Square [78] and Heather was a
frequent visitor from about 1910. At this time the
business was expanding internationally and by 1915
there were Lucile shops in New York, Chicago and
Paris. The shop in Hanover Square was decorated, in
keeping with Duff-Gordon's philosophy for all her
salons, to resemble a domestic space and to reflect
the delicate femininity of her garments: there were
spaces for playing cards, sipping tea and relaxing.
The large rooms had pale grey walls and carpets to
complement the neutral palette of the clothes and
the grand ballroom was used as the main showroom.

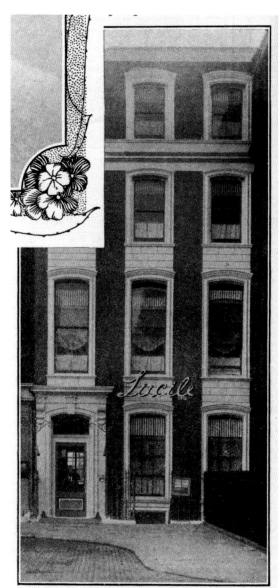

The unpretentious shop whence emanate the wonderful creations
of Lady Duff Gordon   *Photo, Record Press*

Crystal chandeliers, taffeta drapes and silk flowers
added decorative touches and Louis XV chairs were
upholstered in grey silk to match the scheme [80].
Within these grand surroundings, as with all her
salons, a more intimate space, known as the Rose
Room, was created for showing lingerie.[4] Lady Duff-
Gordon remained active throughout the war, particularly in the United States, but afterwards sold her
business. An advertisement in *The Times* on 26 July
1924 shows that the stock of Lucile Ltd of Hanover
Square was to be sold at the Bayswater department
store Whiteley's.

    The Heather Firbank Collection contains 17 Lu-
cile garments, ranging from the delicate 1910 black

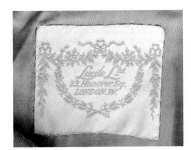

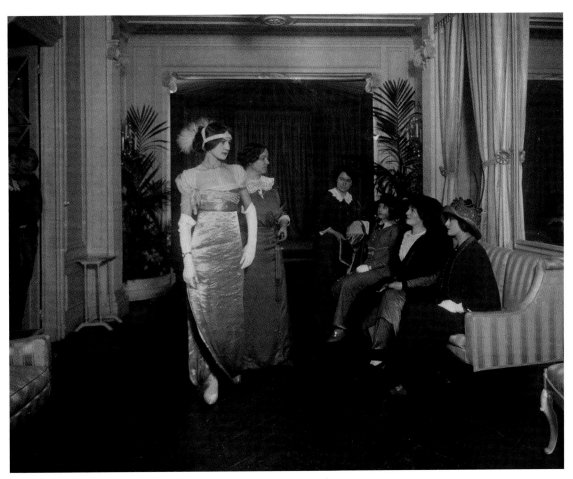

chiffon evening gown to robust tailoring and daywear from during and after the war, together with several bills and other correspondence with the firm, providing a significant body of evidence for Lucile's innovative designs and her contribution to Western fashion. Heather's purple evening dress of 1912 demonstrates Duff-Gordon's ability to translate changing fashions for her English clients. It shows the transition towards the raised waist of the Empire line promoted by Poiret, combined with the rich colours and layers of the tunic style, with a sash and tassel suggesting an opulence inspired by ideas of oriental dress [**83**]. This is an example of an unlabelled Lucile dress, which has the name 'Miss Heather Firbank' written in pencil inside the waistband, in the distinctive hand of a saleswoman or fitter at the fashion house. Other Lucile dresses are marked with Heather's name in exactly the same way, indicating that the completion of Heather's commissions was managed by an individual member of staff who may have been her main point of contact with the firm. Heather was photographed wearing this by Rita Martin (younger sister of Lallie Charles, who took her earlier portraits) around 1912 [**81**]. A design for the dress without the sequinned decoration at the bust can be seen in the Lucile archive at the V&A, suggesting that standard designs were altered to suit the particular tastes of individual clients [**82**].

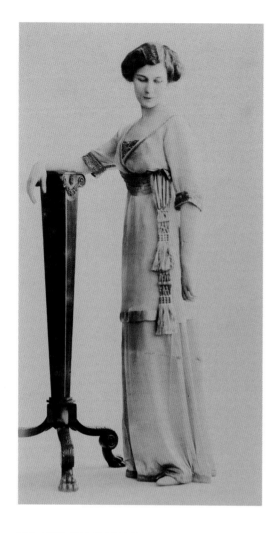

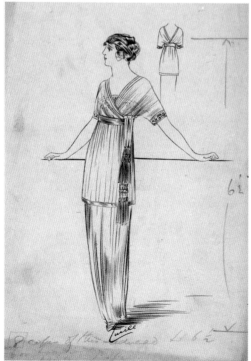

Another Lucile gown of Heather's, an elaborate afternoon dress of ivory satin and silk tulle dating from about 1913, is one of her most fashionable dresses [**84**]. It is trimmed with skunk fur and finished with a wide sash that ties at the back in an enormous showy butterfly bow. The waist is slightly above the natural height and there is a modern-looking asymmetry to the line, with the fur-trimmed ivory chiffon overskirt caught up just off-centre. This layered look became popular around 1912: in this dress three layers are displayed, with the cream machine lace forming an over-tunic, which was sometimes fashioned as a separate garment known as a 'Russian blouse'. The use of machine lace as a key component of fashionable dress was widespread at this time. Handmade lace was used only as a deliberately historical trimming or made by traditional techniques as part of the Arts and Crafts revival. The chiffon and lace overskirts of this dress drape over a tighter inner dress, with the whole lot tapering in at the bottom around the ankles in a shape reminiscent of Poiret's infamous 'hobble' skirt. The wearing of fur reached its heyday in England in the Edwardian era and the fashion continued well into the war years. Worn in both summer and winter for embellishment rather than warmth, it took the form of stoles and large muffs in the earlier years of the century but was worn mainly as trim, as in this example, and as fur coats in the 1910s.[5]

Several other Lucile dresses exemplify a change in Heather's style and display a confidence not seen in the earlier garments in the collection.[6] Her black silk crêpe dinner gown with ivory piping, fashioned in the colours of half-mourning, appropriate for the months following her father's death, is sophisticated and slinky, with a low-cut neckline and the fabric draped to cling to one hip [**85**]. A later cream satin evening dress with black velvet cummerbund also shows a more mature elegance and even sexuality, with the long draped skirt cut with a slit at one side [**87**]. This dress, named 'Eldorado' by Duff-Gordon, was one of several Lucile ensembles included in 'The Secret of Smart Dressing', which shows a mannequin

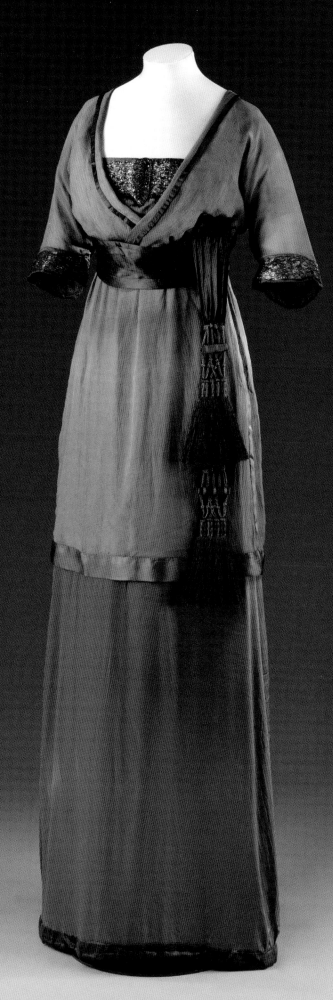

83 Evening dress, silk, silk chiffon and silk satin, embroidered with metal thread and sequins, with silk tassel, Lucile, London, 1912

V&A: T.35-1960

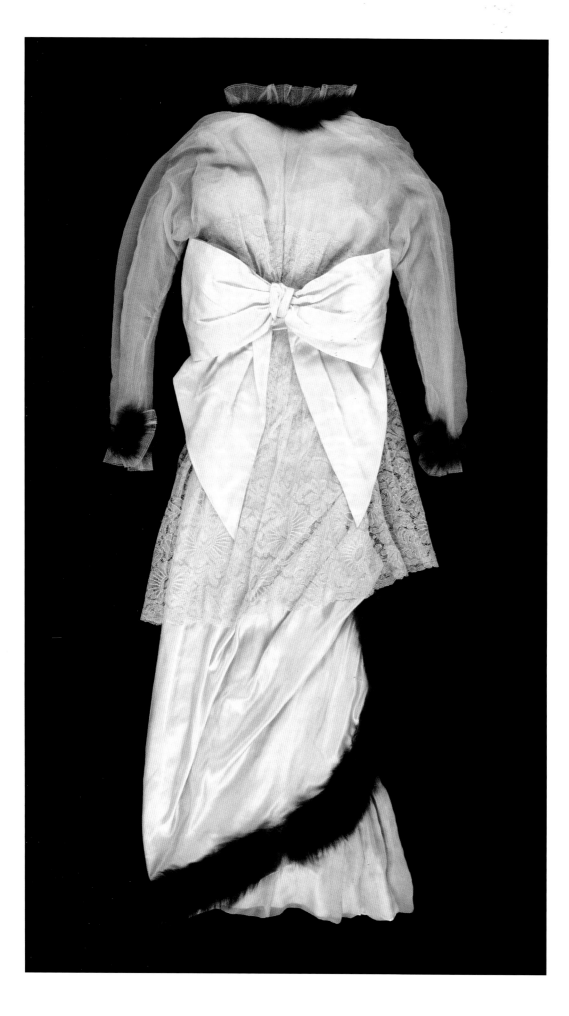

84 Afternoon dress (back view), silk satin, silk chiffon, machine lace, trimmed with skunk fur, Lucile, London, *c.*1913
V&A: T.34–1960

85 Dinner dress, wool crêpe with machine lace insert, edged with silk banding, Lucile, London, *c.*1912
V&A: CIRC.645–1964

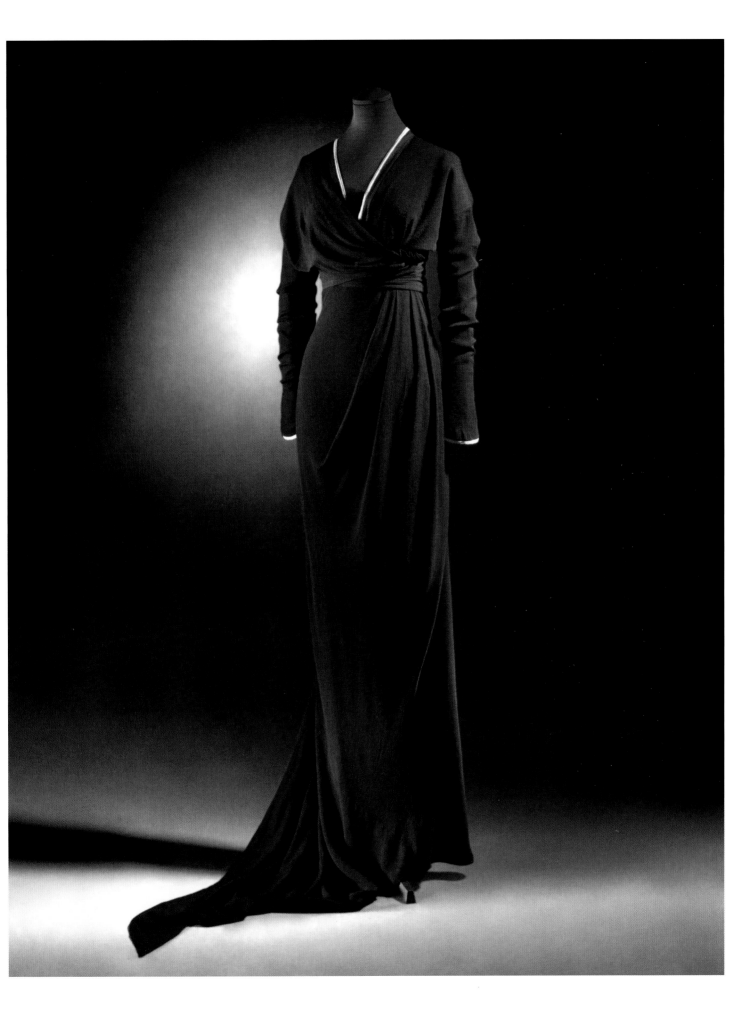

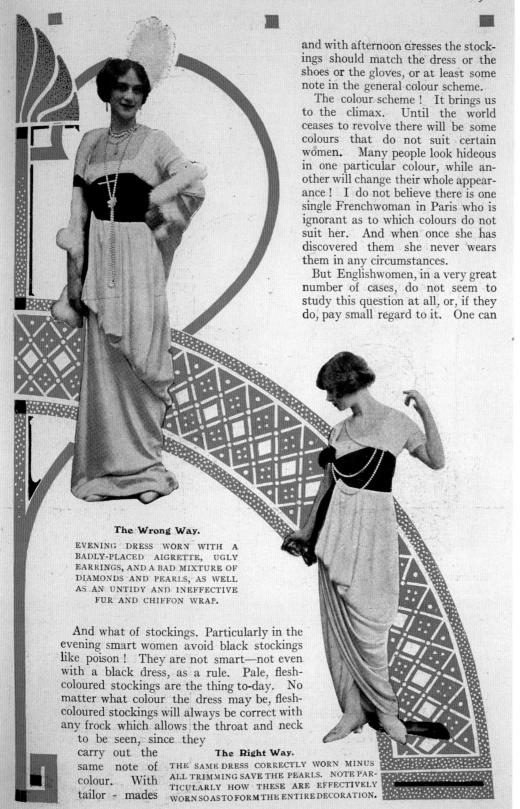

and with afternoon dresses the stockings should match the dress or the shoes or the gloves, or at least some note in the general colour scheme.

The colour scheme! It brings us to the climax. Until the world ceases to revolve there will be some colours that do not suit certain women. Many people look hideous in one particular colour, while another will change their whole appearance! I do not believe there is one single Frenchwoman in Paris who is ignorant as to which colours do not suit her. And when once she has discovered them she never wears them in any circumstances.

But Englishwomen, in a very great number of cases, do not seem to study this question at all, or, if they do, pay small regard to it. One can

The Wrong Way.

EVENING DRESS WORN WITH A BADLY-PLACED AIGRETTE, UGLY EARRINGS, AND A BAD MIXTURE OF DIAMONDS AND PEARLS, AS WELL AS AN UNTIDY AND INEFFECTIVE FUR AND CHIFFON WRAP.

And what of stockings. Particularly in the evening smart women avoid black stockings like poison! They are not smart—not even with a black dress, as a rule. Pale, flesh-coloured stockings are the thing to-day. No matter what colour the dress may be, flesh-coloured stockings will always be correct with any frock which allows the throat and neck to be seen, since they carry out the same note of colour. With tailor - mades

The Right Way.

THE SAME DRESS CORRECTLY WORN MINUS ALL TRIMMING SAVE THE PEARLS. NOTE PARTICULARLY HOW THESE ARE EFFECTIVELY WORN SO AS TO FORM THE ENTIRE DECORATION.

86 'The Secret of Smart Dressing', *The Strand*, December 1913
BRITISH LIBRARY

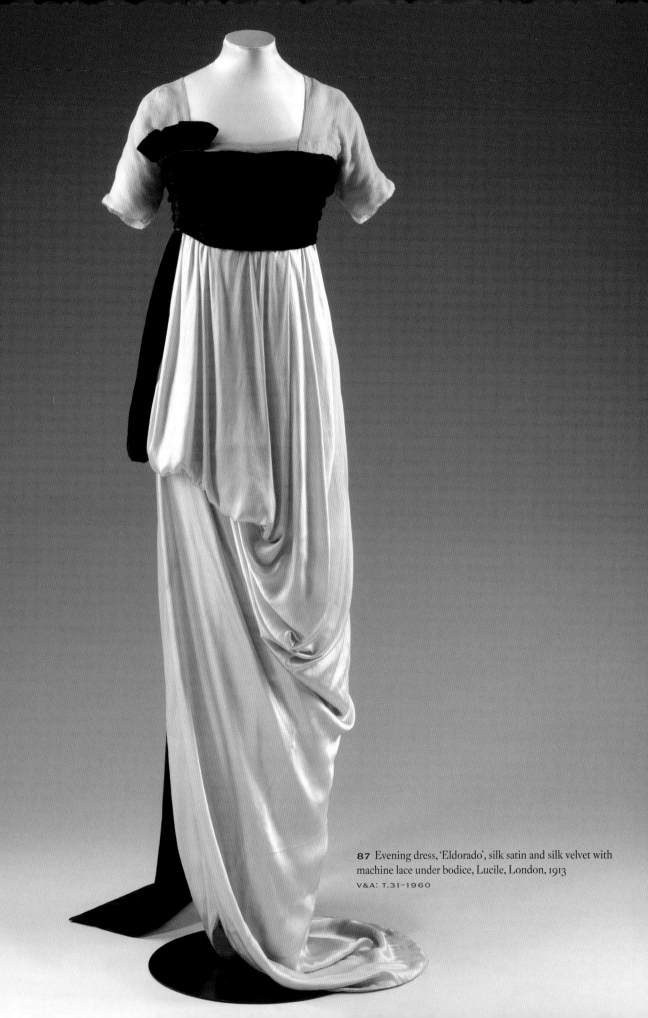

87 Evening dress, 'Eldorado', silk satin and silk velvet with machine lace under bodice, Lucile, London, 1913

V&A: T.31-1960

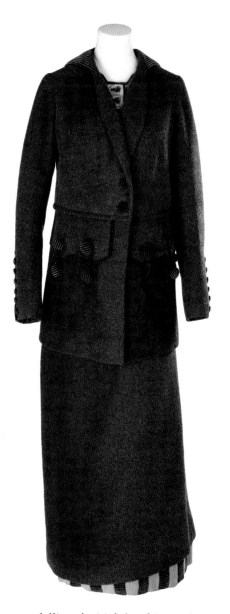

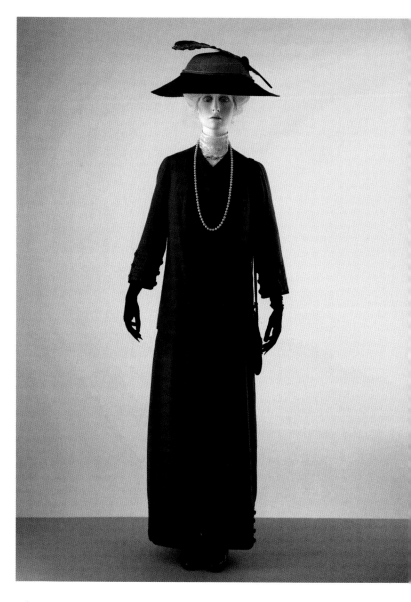

modelling the 'right' and 'wrong' ways to wear the dress and what to wear with it [86].[7] Heather's daywear from this period, again largely purchased from Lucile, is also bravely fashion-conscious. Her charcoal-grey mohair tailored jacket and skirt of 1911 is straighter and more masculine in style than the earlier garments, with bold stripes used as a motif throughout and highly decorative oversized fastenings on the pockets at the front [88]. Another of her Lucile costumes of a similar loose and more masculine shape, with asymmetrical detailing, can be dated precisely to 1912 by a matching design that survives in the Lucile archive [89, 90].

HEATHER'S INDISCRETION

Heather had not met a suitable husband in the two seasons since her presentation at court. For a woman of her wealth, beauty and social position, not to have married is unusual. As Cynthia Asquith reflected in her memoirs: 'Girls were put over the same stiff course again and again, until they married, or, after an untold number of years, officially became Old Maids.'[8] Heather's single status may have been her chosen path, but letters in the collection point to events at this time that would have had a catastrophic impact on the likelihood of her making an advantageous marriage.

An unmarried young woman such as Heather would have lived at home until her wedding day. Her public behaviour was circumscribed by a series of long-established social 'conventions and rules'.

88 Tailored jacket and skirt, wool and mohair with striped silk velvet trim, Lucile, London, 1911

V&A: T.36&A-1960

89 Tailored jacket and skirt, worsted wool, Lucile, London, 1912

V&A: T.38&A-1960

90 Design for Lucile tailored jacket and skirt (see plate 89), Lucile, London, 1912

V&A: LUCILE ARCHIVE, AAD 2008/6/23

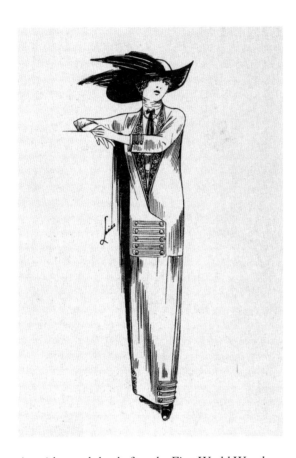

Asquith noted that before the First World War the

chief convention was the indispensability of a chaperone in any public place. To be seen at a theatre, a picture gallery, a restaurant or in a hansom cab alone with a young man was tantamount to announcing your engagement to him or openly advertising that you had decided to throw your cap over the windmill.

She added that she was 'never, never' allowed to go in a train alone. 'I travelled as irresponsibly as a piece of luggage.' She remembered too that 'just to be seen smoking or out alone with a young man was quite enough' for a young woman to be thereafter labelled 'fast' or 'dashing', making it clear how 'easy it was then for girls who liked to "get themselves talked about" to gratify this modest ambition'.[9]

Such an environment makes Heather's choices at this time all the more surprising. At the age of 22, just after her father's death, Heather broke all the rules by conducting an affair with the wealthy aristocrat and MP Colonel William Mitford, who had a distinguished military career. A number of love letters from Mitford survive, dating roughly from 1910 to 1912, written on small sheets of bright blue Pitshill House stationery. The letters are tender and affectionate, but also furtive and secretive, with references to not 'raising suspicions' and burning her letters on receipt. Mitford was 20 years older than Heather and, unfortunately for her, already married.

In such a closely supervised life, conducting a love affair took a great deal of effort. Despite his infatuation, Colonel Mitford remained constantly vigilant about the need for secrecy. The lovers were both members of private clubs in London which served as centres for the exchange of love letters and the arrangement of assignations. Women's clubs, which were established from about the 1880s, provided meals and accommodation for middle-class women and were a safe haven where they could meet like-minded women in central London. The University Club for Ladies, for example, was founded in 1886 as a meeting place for women educated at Oxford and Cambridge. The Grosvenor Crescent Club, founded in 1897, was for professional working women, while the Writers' Club was founded in 1892 at Norfolk Street, just off the Strand.[10]

In 1910–11, Heather was a member of the Ladies' Imperial Club at 17 Dover Street, just three streets away from her family home in Curzon Street. Mitford's equivalent poste restante was the well-established Arthur's Club, just a stone's throw away at 69 St James's Street. An article entitled 'Women's Clubs, Truths from Inside by a Club Woman' in the *Girl's Own Paper Annual* for 1911–12 reveals a widespread mistrust of women's clubs and was deeply critical of the fusion of pretension, shabbiness and feminism to be found in them, while admitting that such clubs offered a service of real value to

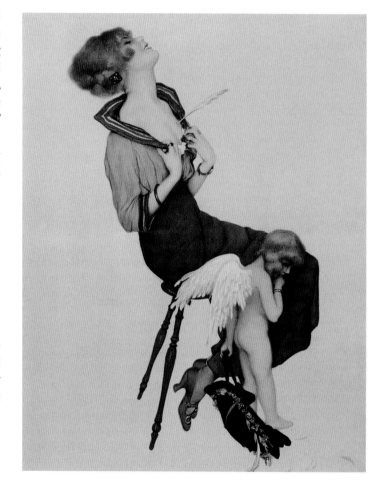

'impecunious members – the women of no special place or position in the world, who are keeping up all the appearance that they can'.[11] Still in mourning for her brother and father, and with Ronald away and no father to control her, Heather perhaps felt alone, with no position in the world. She found refuge and her own poste restante address at the Ladies' Imperial Club.

Although apparently long-lasting in its effect, the romance was short-lived. By 23 June 1911, Colonel Mitford had determined to end the affair, writing:

It really is impossible – We must not meet again ... I cannot go on deceiving C. like this any longer, I have felt so for some time ... If I meet you again my resolution would vanish and that must not be. Let us be friends as before and forget this brief madness, as it truly is. I shall always care for you, dear ... I shall never forget. My love again, Will.[12]

The love affair finally ended around 1912, and a report in the *Daily Express* 'In Society' column dated 24 April of that year suggests that Heather, whether through stress or poor health, was in need of time away from London society. It reads:

Lady Firbank has been most anxious about her only daughter, who has been lying very ill at her brother's house in Curzon Street for several weeks. Miss Heather Firbank has now been ordered by her doctor to leave town for some months' complete rest in the country.[13]

Three further very short letters, which Heather kept and stored, indicate that despite her misfortune with William Mitford she did not lose her ability to attract keen admirers. She moved on to another, briefer love affair, this time with a Frenchman. Just a few lines are written hastily in French on pale blue paper in green ink with an indecipherable signature. The envelopes reveal that these were hand-delivered to her club and came with no return address. The letters are passionate outpourings of his affections, but nonetheless it seems that the affair with Mitford was

still casting a shadow. One letter reads: 'My adored one ... do you really love me or are you trying to forget somebody else?'[14]

Upper-class circles turned a blind eye to extra-marital relations between married people, so had Heather been married herself an affair would have been acceptable, as long as she had provided 'an heir and a spare'. A passage from Vita Sackville-West's *The Edwardians* highlights the normality of this in its account of preparations for a country house weekend: 'This question of the disposition of bedrooms always gave the duchess and her fellow-hostesses cause for anxious thought. It was so necessary to be tactful, and at the same time discreet ... there were recognized lovers to be considered.'[15] Not protected by these social norms as a young unmarried woman, however, Heather was extremely vulnerable. It is not clear whether her affairs ever became public knowledge, but had they been discovered, her reputation would have been in tatters.

Looking at Heather's wardrobe from this period, these love affairs seem to coincide with the adoption of a slightly more risqué style: her choices became bolder, more highly fashionable and more alluring, though they remained within conventional boundaries. The wearing of deliberately nonconformist styles of dress, particularly by young society women but also by young men, was clear public defiance of social norms and was practised before the First World War only by women such as Ottoline Morrell, Vanessa Bell and Dorelia John, who set out to create such identities for themselves. Through her brother Ronald, with his extremely dandified appearance and his acquaintances within bohemian and gay circles, Heather was close to nonconformist dressers, but she chose to take no part in their social world.

HEATHER AND RONALD

Heather and her older brother were close throughout their lives [92]. Ronald suffered from asthma and weak lungs and spent much of his time travelling abroad 'for the better climate', writing to Heather ('Baby') and his mother ('Baba') almost daily. He recommended books for Heather to read and she kept him up to date with the latest fashions.

Ronald was an eccentric. Osbert Sitwell, who was at Cambridge with him and knew him as well as anybody could know such a 'paralysingly shy' man, described him as having 'a taste for the exotic', being 'fond of smart society' but 'a fantasist ... not like others' and a writer in the 'experiment of artificial comedy' [93].[16] Had unmarried Heather belonged to the world of bohemia like her brother, a world which despised the rules of conventional 'respectable' society for women and in which her brother spent most of his life – in London, Rome, Paris, the

Middle East and North Africa – her love affair would not have mattered even before the First World War. This was the world of Nancy Cunard, Nina Hamnett, Augustus John and Wyndham Lewis, and Ronald knew them all. Heather, in her elegant London couture clothes, was of course very far from a bohemian, in either her dress or her relationships, and there is no evidence that she ever met Ronald's bohemian friends or shared his bohemian outlook.

When three of Ronald's novels [94] were reissued in 2012, writer and journalist Philip Womack described them as 'weirdly fluid tableaux studded with jewels, full of peacocks, laughter and hidden sadness; oblique, glancing, beams of sunlight trapped in glass. His characters are effete, idle, existing in a world where art is effectively life.'[17] Womack added that the frivolity in Ronald's writing was in fact 'eminently serious' and that without him 'we would not have had

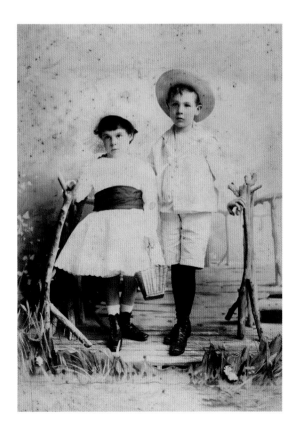

Aldous Huxley, Evelyn Waugh or Henry Green. His ultimate descendant is William Burroughs.'[18]

Although they did not share the same social scene, Heather and Ronald were both passionate about clothes. Ronald took great care in his appearance [**95**]. Patricia Juliana Smith writes: 'Like many introverts, he compensated for social inadequacies through eccentricities and his extraordinary dandyism.'[19] He worried, as his sister did not, about the cost of his new clothes when ordering bespoke tailoring for his rare visits to London in the 1920s. He wrote to Heather that his tailoring bills made such London visits 'expensive [because of] clothes I need after so long'. Despite this concern, he nevertheless ordered his Savile Row suits from one of London's most famous tailoring establishments, Henry Poole.[20]

Ronald spent years scolding his sister for overspending on couture gowns while at the same time understanding her passion for them. His writings reflect this interest, with characters sumptuously described in fantastically fashionable clothing. The character of the Baroness in *The Artificial Princess* is described as:

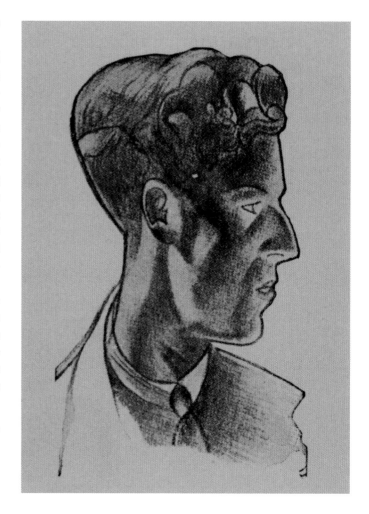

looking angelic in a gown of three shades of grey, with silver embroideries and improvised knots and falling tassels, partly concealing the 'heavenly aquarelles', which was perhaps just as well. Quantities of tiny painted buttons ran hither and thither, quite aimlessly, going nowhere, all undone. Like yellow butterflies the Winged Victories hovered from her ears, and a string of filmy stones, obviously spells, peeped furtively, like watchful eyes, waiting to operate at a moment's warning, in ways best known to themselves. She was looking pale, and unusually weary, under an enormous structure of feathers and orchids, weighed down on one side in artistic collapse. In her delicate Greco hands, cased in stiff white kid, she carried the frailest of wicker baskets and tucked under her arm an elaborate sunshade of geranium pink.[21]

Ronald's novels make reference to Heather's favourite dressmakers, including Lucile and Redfern.[22] His descriptions reflect the luxurious clothing in his sister's wardrobe and the attention to detail and fastidious research behind her clothing choices.

Heather's interest in fashion never left her, despite the family's increasingly straitened circumstances. On 13 September 1919, Lady Firbank begged Heather:

not to spend a penny you can avoid. Should you get in debt again it will then be absolutely out of my power to clear you or even to help to do so – I am sure the luncheons you had from Harrods last time you were up, at £1.17.0 were not necessary and lots of things you get there ... [you] could do without.

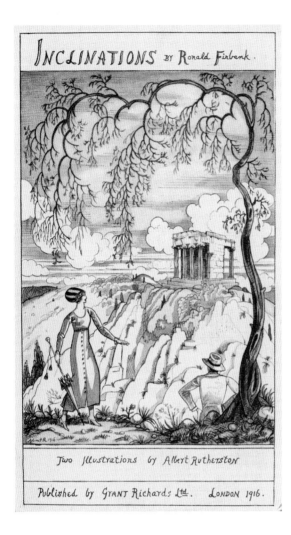

94 Advertisement for *Inclinations* by Ronald Firbank, illustrated by Albert Rutherston, England, 1916
V&A: E.2459-1953

95 Ronald Firbank in Chamonix, France, 1904

She added that after her own death Heather would receive an annuity of £525.[23] Three years later Heather had so dramatically overspent her allowance that her mother was reduced to suggesting to Ronald that some of the family's remaining silver ornaments could be sold to pay off her debts. Ronald wrote to his mother exasperatedly from Fiesole on 5 April 1922:

It is very sad to have so squandered everything. I do think it imprudent to sell silver which we may need to sell in illness or emergency, to meet these dressmakers' bills! I should part with nothing if you can avoid it.[24]

'YOU ARE MY ONLY BROTHER. I HAVE NO ONE LEFT BUT YOURSELF' [25]

For many of those coming of age in the early twentieth century it was the impact of the First World War that brought about the change in their lives. For Heather, however, personal choices and family misfortune in the pre-war years had the most profound impact on her adulthood. Following the untimely deaths of her brother Joey in 1904 and her father in 1910, Heather's youngest brother, Hubert, unexpectedly succumbed to illness and died aged just 25 in 1913. Hubert ('Bertie') had been living in Canada since 1909 with his wife and young son, Thomas, born in 1910. Thomas, Heather's only nephew, had two daughters and is the father of Johanna Firbank, the last surviving member of the Firbank family. With Bertie's death, Heather and Ronald were left as the only two surviving Firbank siblings and grew increasingly reliant on each other. The death of her father and two brothers, the loss of the family's money, and the decision to carry on a love affair with a married man of status and wealth meant that Heather entered her late twenties during Britain's most catastrophic conflict to date in the shadow of depression and in a position of dwindling status and questionable reputation.

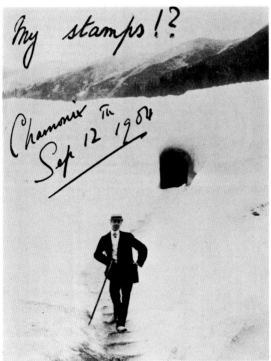

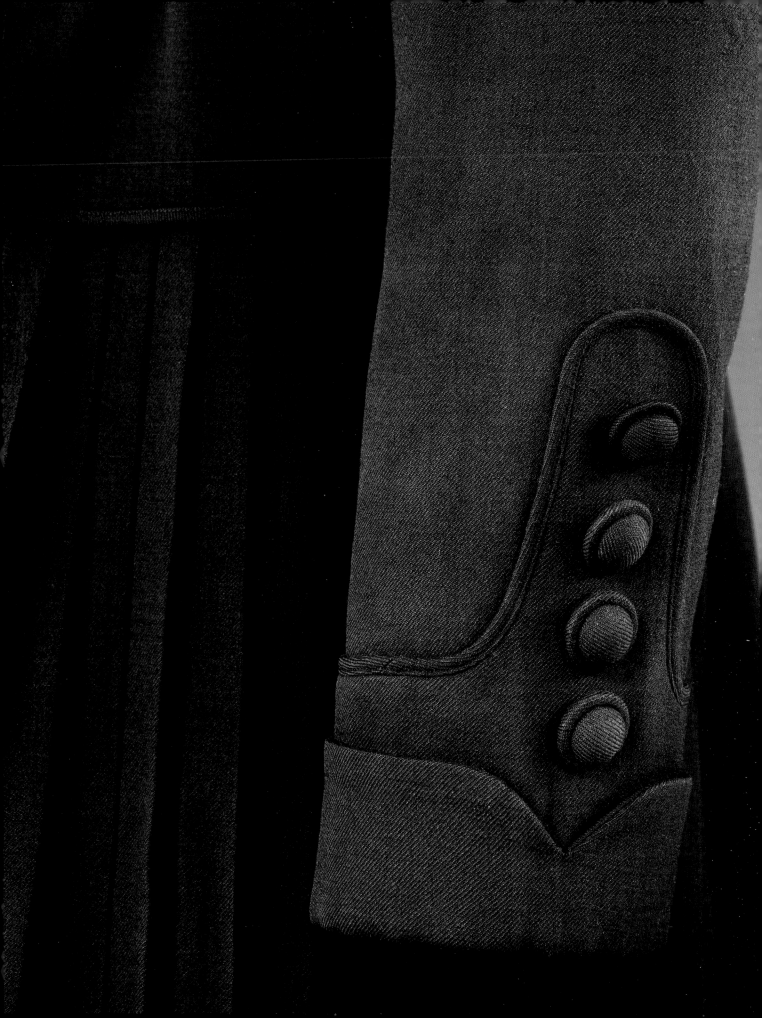

WARTIME AND AFTER:
A RETREAT FROM SOCIETY
1914–24

Britain declared war on 4 August 1914, marking the start of four years of intensive fighting for the country. The enormous loss of life on the battlefields was not reflected in Heather's immediate experience of the war, nor was the clothing industry affected in the way it would be during the Second World War, with the impact of rationing. The world of fashion in London and Paris continued to develop, and journalists dutifully reported the changes. On 11 July 1914, a fortnight after the assassination of Archduke Franz Ferdinand and his wife, the 'Fashion Forecast' section of *The Queen* announced:

[A]s even the least intelligent must be aware, we are walking on very shifting sands; great radical changes are taking place alike in silhouette and the general acceptance of what constitutes elegance.

We are making surely and steadily … for a more harmonious simplicity. We have worked eccentricity and extravagance to a thread, and … changes have been brought about in a few months that would heretofore have taken at least two, if not three, years to be worked up into acceptance.[1]

Fashions fluctuated between pared-down sombre-looking garments and full-colour, full-skirted ensembles, reflecting the uncertainty of the times [100]. The general shift was towards a rising hemline and greater simplicity, ultimately leading to the birth of the modern wardrobe. Heather's surviving wartime outfits, worn when she was in her late twenties, include sober tailor-made costumes, a plain blue linen summer dress and coats with bold abstract details. The collection also includes a few items from the early 1920s. The two most striking features of this later clothing are the lack of evening wear, unusual for a woman of her age, and the lack

of colour, reflecting her changing circumstances.

With no immediate family in military service, Heather and her mother lived out the war years in an apartment in Sloane Street. Heather's papers indicate that, like many women of her background, she had an interest in doing war work, and she wrote to a cousin asking for contacts in the Foreign Office, intending to seek employment. She received a reply on 25 August 1918, two and a half months before the war ended, suggesting that it 'would be a pity' if her 'language proficiency was wasted', but it seems that ultimately nothing came of these efforts.[2]

Although she was not directly involved with the war, profound changes were taking place in Heather's personal life. By the age of 26, she had lost three close family members and had been devastated by an ultimately fruitless love affair which had consumed her early twenties. From the surviving letters between her and Ronald it seems that this deep loss had left her exhausted and depressed and, with no independent income, increasingly isolated. Without either the means or the inclination to travel, despite frequent suggestions from her brother, she continued to buy her clothes from the places she trusted and knew best. As the bills from Lucile testify, despite dwindling funds she continued with her established extravagant purchasing patterns.

'THE MUCH TALKED-OF MILITARY NOTE'
Though Heather's clothes from this period were more subdued, they continued to be well made and stylish, reflecting the changing shape of fashionable dress to the more boyish silhouette and shorter hemlines of the 1920s. Three ensembles in Heather's wardrobe

96 Tailored jacket (detail of plate 99)

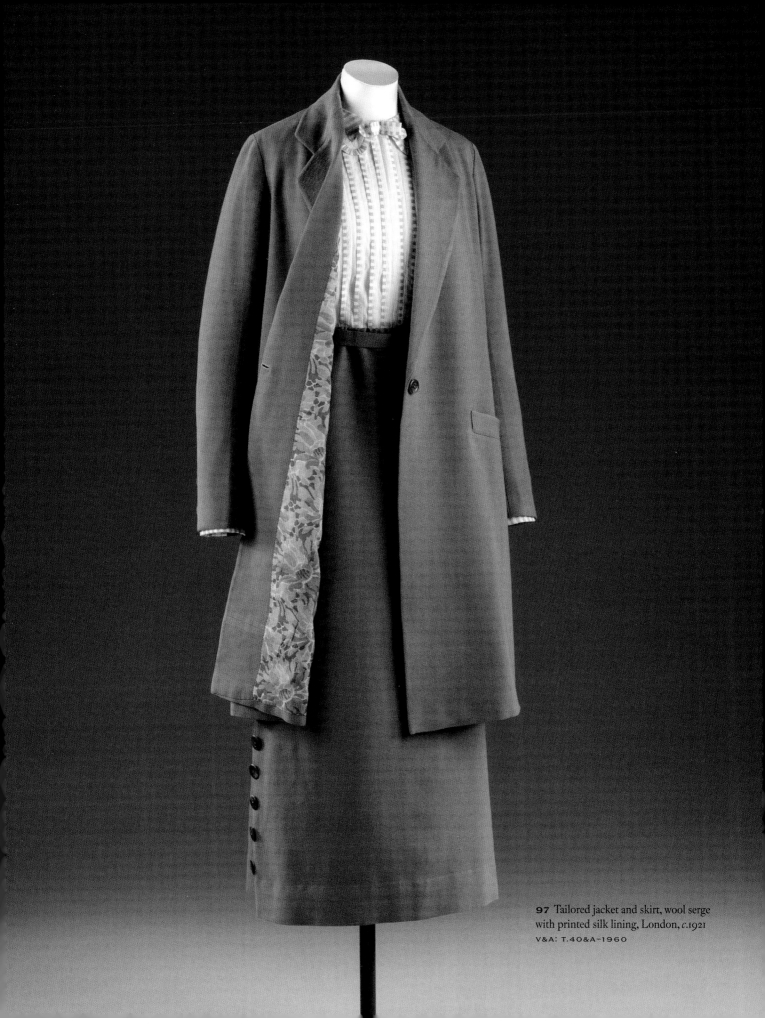

97 Tailored jacket and skirt, wool serge
with printed silk lining, London, *c.*1921
V&A: T.40&A–1960

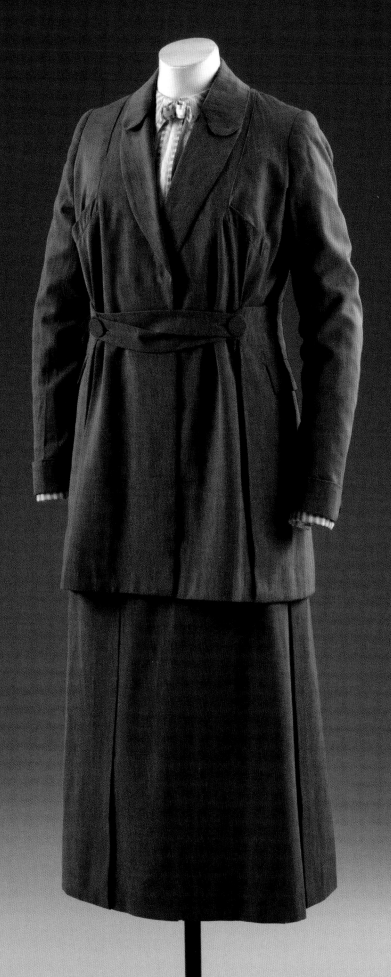

98 Tailored jacket and skirt, silk
and wool, Lucile, London, *c.*1917
V&A: T.41&A-1960

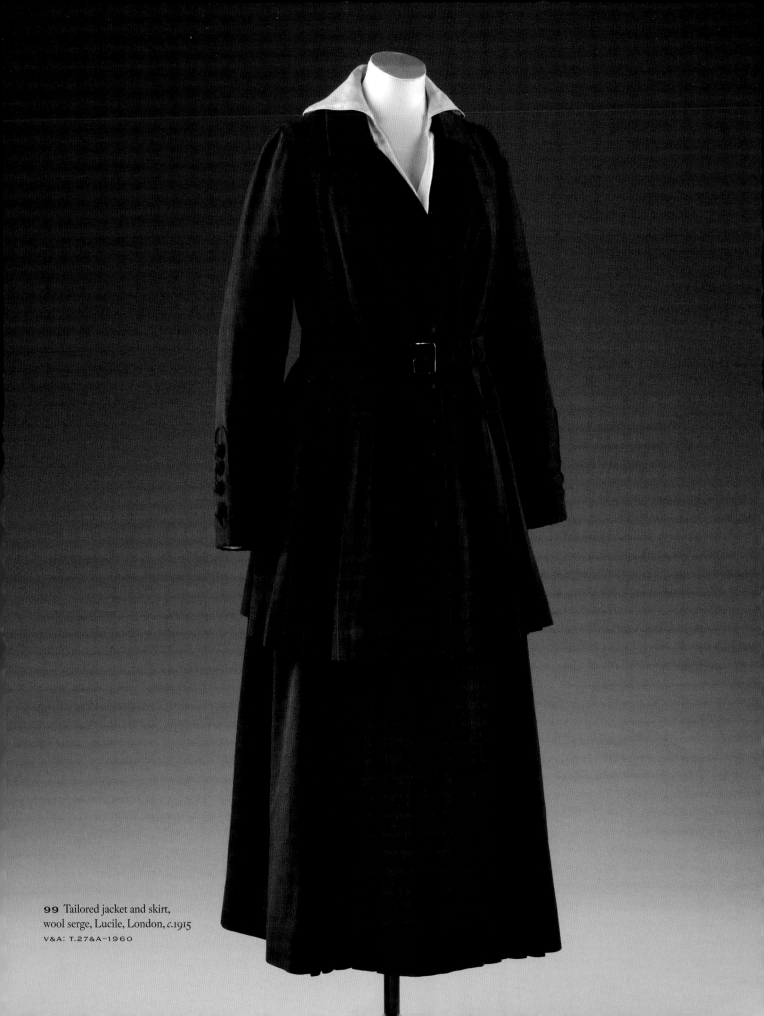

99 Tailored jacket and skirt,
wool serge, Lucile, London, *c*.1915
V&A: T.27&A-1960

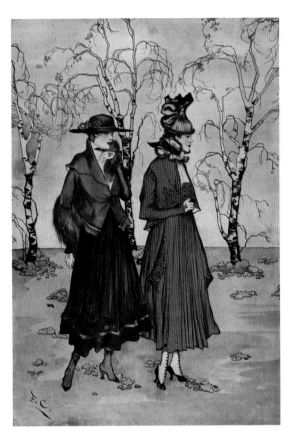

colour and style, of a military garment [**98**]. Another tailored costume, in navy-blue/black, also from Lucile and from around the same time, shows a hint of the fuller shape that was in vogue in its pleated skirt, but could arguably also show military influence in the belted jacket and the positioning of the buttons and detailing around the cuffs [**99**]. Belted coats such as these were sometimes referred to as 'sports coats' and are arguably simpler and less restrictive than the tailored costumes of the 1900s. A long plain beige wool jacket and mid-length skirt from the early 1920s shows the movement towards even greater simplicity [**97**]. It is loose-fitting and closes with a single button at the front. The only decoration is provided by lines of buttons trimming the sides of the skirt, the cuffs and the open sides of the jacket. This costume is not labelled, but, as with her earlier purchases, Heather has chosen a bold lining for the jacket, faced with colourful floral silk, which was very fashionable at the time and which continued to be popular to the end of the 1920s.

A blue linen day dress of Heather's shows the shorter hemline in dresses with a skirt that falls well above the ankle [**101**]. Although finely made, the fabric, simple shape and deep pockets give the dress a utilitarian look. The polka-dot silk bow at the front is the only trimming. The bodice is not boned, but it is firmly anchored at the waist with a deep internal waistband; it closes with a short line of hooks and eyes along the inner layer and practical, easy-to-close metal poppers on the outer layer. Although still challenging to put on without help, it is far simpler than the 30 hooks and eyes on the Edwardian pink linen day dress of less than 10 years earlier [see **28**].

With looser-fitting forms around the waist, corsets were no longer required to shape the figure quite so dramatically. They became shorter, concentrating on the lower torso, and with the growing popularity of dancing they became less heavily boned and more elasticated to allow greater movement. Heather owned what became known as a 'tango' corset, bought

from about 1915 to 1921 show the changes in tailored costumes. The influence of military clothing on wartime high fashion, visible in these tailor-mades, has been much debated, and it seems that this was also the case for contemporary observers. A fashion commentator in *The Queen* wrote in November 1914:

The much talked-of military note in dress does not impress me mightily. There is, true enough, a certain element pervading both millinery and modes that is loosely described as military ... Of the loose application then we have an apt illustration in the familiar wide, low-belted coat, which may be verily said to have almost entirely shouldered out the flowing cavalier cape of spring. Why in the name of sense this coat is so frequently invested with military titles, such as the 'Cossack', 'Guards', or just simply defined as Military, it yet remains to be found out.

There is ... little ... to warrant the word military being dragged in ... Name it how you like, the model stands finely representative of the correct silhouette of the hour.[3]

Heather had two such low-belted tailored costumes from Lucile. One is of light brown wool serge and has an overlapping belt which closes with two buttons at the back and front and does have the feel, in

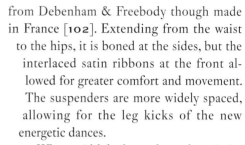

101 Summer day dress, linen, silk organza, silk ribbon, British, *c.*1915
V&A: T.17–1960

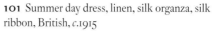

from Debenham & Freebody though made in France [**102**]. Extending from the waist to the hips, it is boned at the sides, but the interlaced satin ribbons at the front allowed for greater comfort and movement. The suspenders are more widely spaced, allowing for the leg kicks of the new energetic dances.

Where width had once been the priority in millinery, height now became of interest, with smaller hats supporting towering trimmings, such as tall waving ostrich feathers, or 'willow plumes' as they were known. Heather's dramatic monochrome example pairs a deep cloche-style black straw hat wrapped in black waxed ribbon with a large white ostrich feather, extended at the tip with a fine egret feather of very pale pink [see **58**]. An illustration of Ranelagh polo from the *Illustrated London News* in June 1914 shows the popularity of this brief trend [**106**]. Brochures in the collection from Nice Ostrich Farm show that Heather bought feathers direct from them to retrim her hats when they became tired. This would have been another skill her lady's maid, Hallett, had to perfect.

Many patterns of social and fashionable behaviour that had been fundamental among the upper classes before the war seemed outmoded and frivolous in wartime and after. With the greater simplicity in dress came a paring down of the range of garments needed throughout the day. Tailored costumes, which had long been a staple of a woman's daytime wardrobe, were adapted for evening wear with the introduction of matching dresses and jackets. Heather owned a strikingly modern-looking example by Lucile in navy-blue serge with a mandarin collar and black piping trimming. The dress would have been worn with

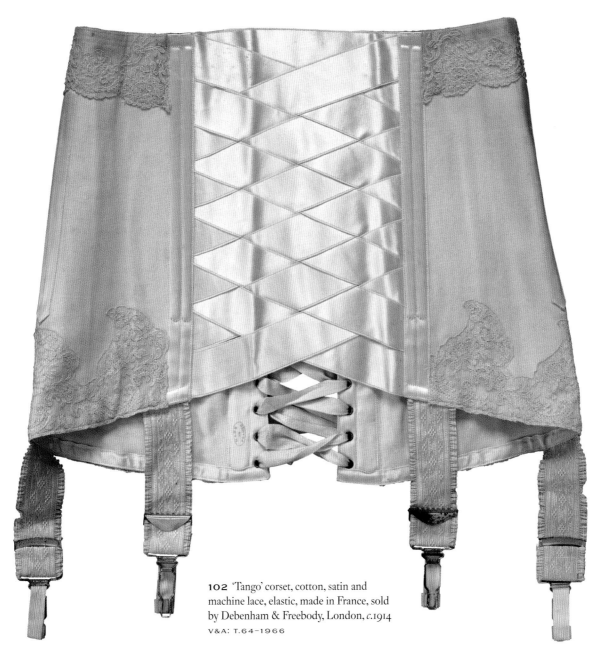

102 'Tango' corset, cotton, satin and machine lace, elastic, made in France, sold by Debenham & Freebody, London, c.1914
V&A: T.64-1966

the collarless jacket during the day and the jacket removed later to reveal the matching mid-calf dress for informal dining, which has black satin sleeves and a belted waist [105]. The use of black trimmings and fabrics combined with navy-blue serge in this outfit repeats a recurrent theme in Heather's wardrobe, seen in earlier tailor-made costumes from Redfern [see 32].

The latest garment in the Heather Firbank Collection, which dates from the mid-1920s, is a light summer day dress of striped silk with a built-in blouse. Easy to put on and comfortable to wear, it is typical of the greater freedom seen in women's clothing in the new decade [103].

MY HEALTH SEEMS BROKEN ...

As Ronald was already spending most of his time abroad and there were no social reasons for the widowed Lady Firbank to retain her central London property, Ronald disposed of the Belgravia apartment in 1919, setting up his mother and sister in Denbigh Cottage, a rented house in Richmond.[4] They moved there with some of the remaining late-eighteenth-century furniture, Heather's piano and some of their porcelain and silver pieces, dropping further out of the London social scene. This represented a significant loss in status for the family, who had always had a presence in central London. From this point on Heather began a new chapter, leaving

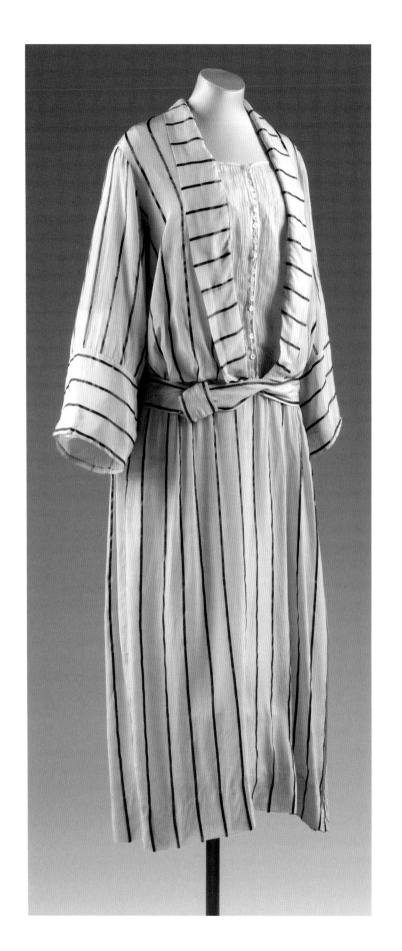
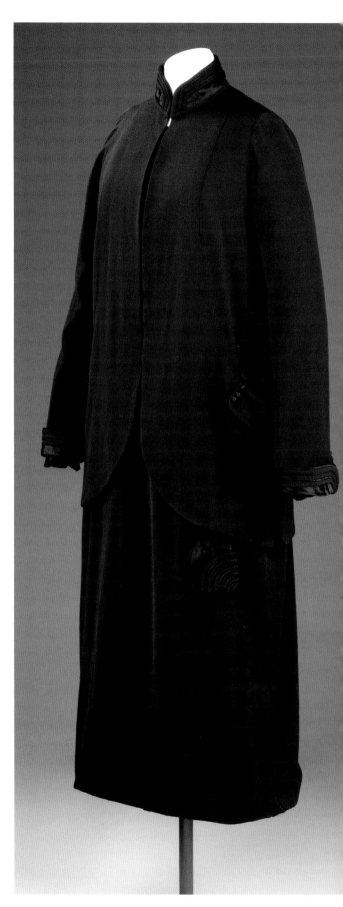

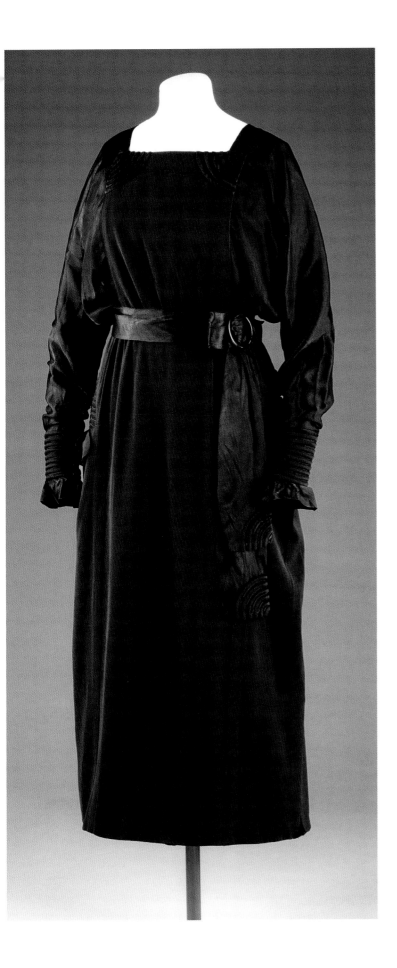

103 Summer day dress, striped silk, British, 1920–25
V&A: T.19–1960

104 Tailored dress and jacket, wool serge, satin, Lucile, London, *c*.1915
V&A: T.50&A–1960

105 Tailored dress, wool serge, satin, Lucile, London, *c*.1915
V&A: T.50–1960

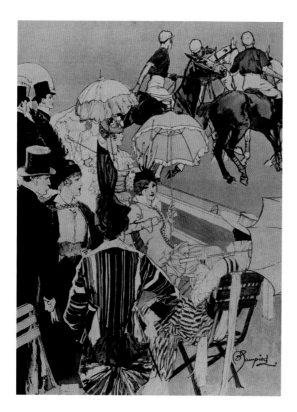

106 Polo at Ranelagh, *Illustrated London News*, June 1914
V&A: NAL

107 Evening dress, silk with silk velvet appliqué and metal thread embroidery, Myrbor, Paris, *c.*1923, worn by Emilie Grigsby
V&A: CIRC.329-1968

society life behind and retreating to a quieter, more isolated existence in Richmond.

Her wardrobe, with its lack of evening wear from this time, reflects the change. Hallett was retained as housekeeper. A car was kept and a chauffeur hired because Heather, now no longer able to walk from her home to her favourite couturiers, required private transport into central London. Just two years after the move to Richmond, she wrote a letter to her brother that revealed how unhappy she was and her desire to find a way out of her isolated situation. In response, Ronald wrote to Heather: 'I certainly think you <u>need</u> a change & should not give up the idea of trying to manage it. Everything I fully realise is very difficult.'[5]

Although Heather's wardrobe follows the key changes in fashion, there is neither the exuberance nor the sense of adventure that is to be seen in some of her contemporaries' wardrobes of the early 1920s. The clothes of the flamboyant and beautiful American Emilie Grigsby, for example, which are in the V&A's collections, reflect her life of foreign travel and socializing as the former lover of the extremely wealthy American businessman Charles T. Yerkes. Grigsby's clothes, mainly purchased from Paris, are full of colour and designed for dancing the new crazes such as the Charleston [107]. In contrast, Heather took little advantage of the greater social

freedoms available to well-off, independent women after the First World War. Instead, between 1920 and 1925, she lived quietly in Richmond, where, with the help of Hallett, she nursed her mother, who was dying of cancer. As Emilie Grigsby's world was opening up, Heather's was closing in, a fact evident in their contrasting wardrobes.

As a single woman in this period, Heather was in a uniquely vulnerable situation, living in 'the shadow of marriage'. This position is underlined by Pat Jalland in her book *Women, Marriage and Politics 1860–1914*, where she writes of unmarried women such as Heather:

They were usually financially dependent on male members of the family – often a sufficient explanation for their exploitation. Their social and economic position was exceptionally vulnerable, for they faced the possible loss of home, status and function in life with the death of a father or the marriage of a brother. Spinsters often had an ill-defined role in the family, with little recognition that they were individuals with interests, needs and identities of their own.[6]

Less than a month after their mother's death in 1924, Ronald wrote to Heather explaining that they would have to give up the lease on Denbigh Cottage and that she would have to leave by the end of the year so that he could sell it. This instruction started a dispute between the two of them that continued for well over a year.[7] Ronald's patience with his sister's spending seems to have reached its limit in February 1925, when he wrote again, saying:

Now as you do not seem to be able to live economically at Denbigh Cottage (You are living at present there at a rate of more than £1000 a year, has it occurred to you?) I feel hardly encouraged to postpone the letting, or the selling of it another year ... your Annuity ... should go towards 'Jones' the greengrocer as well as 'Lucile' the dressmaker – it seems a little <u>stupid</u> to <u>have</u> to point out!!!?[8]

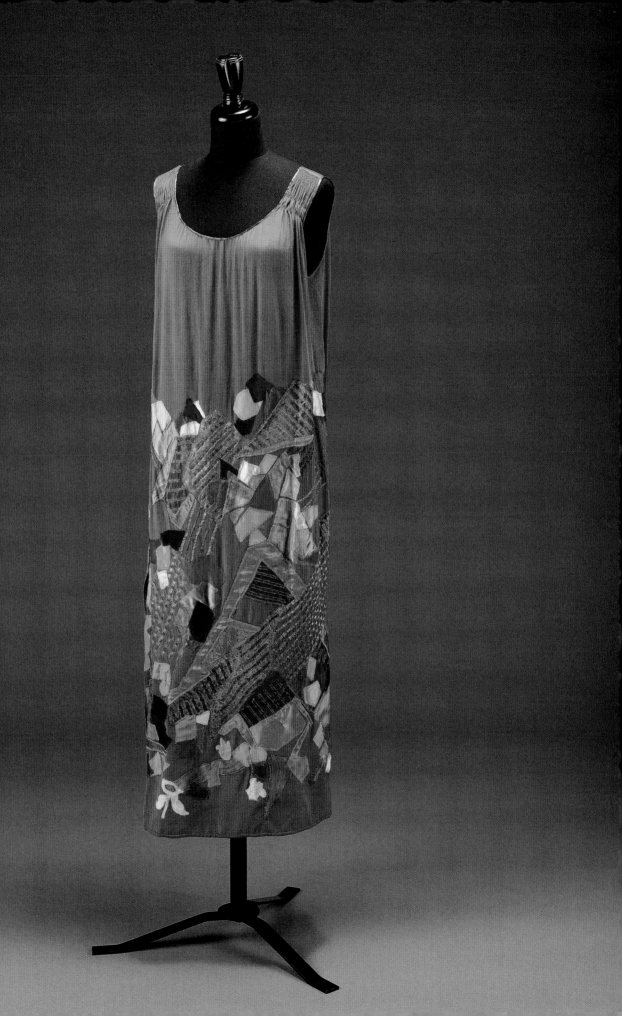

Heather wrote back with increasing desperation a few weeks later:

I cannot bring myself to believe that you remain so indifferent to my extremely difficult position. Let me tell you that I have no alternative but to beg of you to help me & without delay ... I am such a wreck that I am quite unable to undertake the effort of finding a cheap cottage out in the country. My health seems broken and because of that – even were I financially able – to travel as you suggest is absolutely out of the question. What I need is rest – mental and physical after the incessant strain and grief I have been through. Therefore, if you will reconsider & promise to let me return to Denbigh Cottage, any time soon, you will save me a certain breakdown ... I am feeling so ill and so sad.[9]

Despite her pleas, Ronald decided to terminate the lease in Richmond and the siblings became property-less, marking a further loss in status for the Firbanks. Heather eventually moved to a ladies' club in Mayfair, although she continued to plead with her brother to let her stay at Denbigh Cottage. The lease came to an end in 1925 and the two siblings finally settled their differences at the office of their solicitors that same year. While Ronald's decision left his sister homeless

and led to her peripatetic existence thereafter, it did ensure that she was well off. For the remaining years of her life, Heather lived in hotels and rented apartments, dividing her time between London and Sussex.[10]

Ronald took responsibility for Heather emotionally and financially: he arranged her housing and allowance, and extra funding would be permitted with his approval only. The last of Heather's immediate family, he died in Rome on 21 May 1926, aged just 40.[11] That year, Heather put into storage the exquisite collection of clothes which after her own death was offered to the V&A.[12] None of her clothes or photographs survive beyond the mid-1920s, but enough alternative evidence, including account books and letters, still exists, enabling us to build up a picture of the rest of her life.

LATER LIFE

Heather settled in Sussex, a county she knew well. Her mother used to go to Brighton for annual holidays and Heather stayed frequently at Petworth between 1910 and 1912. Family archives show that between about 1933 and 1936 she maintained an independent flat at 2 St Aubyns Mansions, Hove, a street of imposing four-storey mid-Victorian family

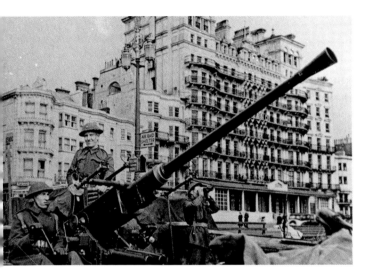

homes close to the seafront. She then lived in some style in a private apartment with a Steinway piano in the Princes Hotel – a grand, luxurious, if by then old-fashioned Victorian establishment on Hove seafront – from 1936 to 1937 [**108**]. In a letter written in February 1932, on Princes Hotel notepaper, Daphne Du Maurier described the hotel to her friend Foy Quiller-Couch:

Pile carpets, central heating, running water in rooms, private bath ... I did not know such people as live here really existed outside French burlesques of 'the English'. Over-fed colonels with swimming stomachs and purple faces, thin tight lipped elderly spinsters. They all talk in whispers or else very loudly suddenly about their health. I suppose they are here because 'abroad' is too expensive. I expect they are the people who have 'made England what it is'. Outposts of the Empire sort of business, and 'the country is going to the dogs sir'. They probably discuss the India question and say with the usual unintelligent pomposity, 'what those native fellows need is a firm hand'. And the spinsters go all bitter and curious when they look at young married women.[13]

Heather continued to spend at luxury stores. Occasionally she purchased from Hanningtons, the most fashionable department store in Brighton, and indeed in Sussex, but it is clear that while living at the Princes Hotel her fashion store of preference was now Bradley's of 1 Chepstow Place, near Westbourne Grove. The company employed 600 staff, including its own in-house fashion designers, and customers included Winston Churchill and his wife, Hollywood film stars and members of the royal family.[14] We do not know what garments Heather selected from this fashionable store for her life in the Princes Hotel but she was spending large amounts of money there – £48 6s on 19 July 1937, a further £78 15s 6d on 17 February 1938 and £150 on 8 May 1939. Heather rarely – indeed, almost never – travelled by public transport, keeping up her mother's tradition of employing a chauffeur to drive a private limousine, probably kept in the hotel's garage.[15]

Heather's life in the Princes Hotel ended abruptly at the start of the Second World War, in September 1939. The entire section of the Hove seafront where Heather was living was taken over by the army and the navy. It was cordoned off with great rolls of barbed wire, with Bofors guns placed at regular intervals along the length of the promenade [**109**]. Streets were blocked to civilians and the hotel was requisitioned by the navy, becoming HMS *Lizard*, a land-based naval centre. There is no evidence that Heather, now in her fifties, took part in any war work during the Second World War. A letter dating from 1943 reveals that she probably spent the war years living in a cottage in Withdean, a quiet area in the north of Brighton.

Heather's last known private address was the County Hotel in Lindfield, 12 miles from Brighton. Finally, ill health forced her into the Brooklands Nursing Home in Haywards Heath. She died there in 1954, aged 67.[16] Her memory lives on in her remarkable collection of clothing at the V&A, which has enriched numerous displays and exhibitions and will continue to do so for generations to come.

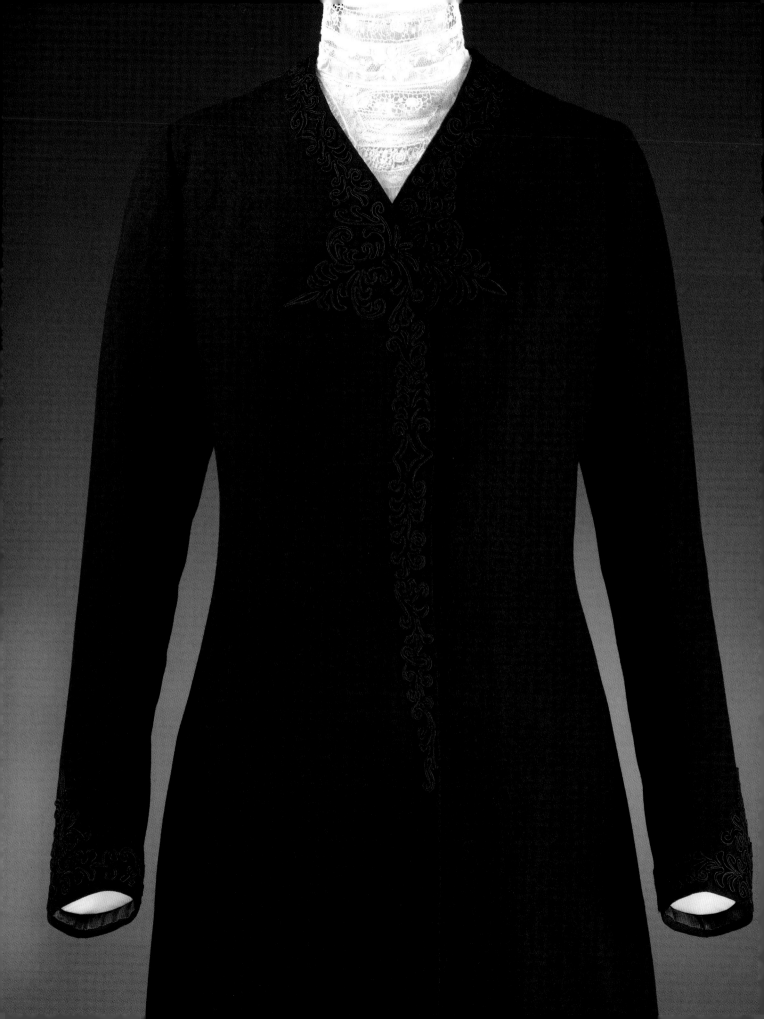

HEATHER FIRBANK AND
LONDON'S COUTURE INDUSTRY

Looking back on London during the period from 1907 until the outbreak of the First World War, Charlotte Mortimer, then a managing director of Worth (London), recalled in the 1950s:

It was one of the most feminine and elegant periods of dress that has ever been ... High fashion was more on view then because women walked far more. They shopped on foot because everything could be ordered and sent and they strolled in the parks and squares. The management of long skirts and accessories like parasols and muffs was looked upon as a real art ... And of course, the hats were enchanting, all flowers and ribbons and veiling ...

'Going to the dressmaker' was looked upon as a social activity, as much a part of the fashionable pattern as the At Home or the dinner party. By five o'clock Hanover Square and the streets all round were filled with waiting carriages and there were usually little groups of spectators waiting to see the notables.[1]

Dressing fashionably, as we have seen, was a serious occupation, a public performance requiring a significant investment of time and expertise. A conventional wealthy upper-class woman expected to devote her energy and her husband's (or father's) financial resources to maintaining the correct appearance. Such complicated wardrobes, which needed to be updated regularly to accommodate changing fashions, different events of the London season, and occasions such as court presentations, weddings, coronations and public mourning, generated a great demand for the specialized skills of workers in the British textile and fashion industries, especially at the height of the London season, from April to August. Well-dressed and fashionable women such as Heather Firbank,

wearing the products of London's department stores and dressmakers' and milliners' shops, were a sign of the British Empire's industrializing and free-trade economy. With numerous fashion magazines and easier transport links to Europe, upper-class English women had increased access to French fashion and wished to be as 'smartly gowned as their Parisian sisters'. In response, London dressmakers adapted and expanded to answer this increased demand, and as one (admittedly British) newspaper reported in 1910: 'There is no occasion to go to Paris for beautiful dresses and to learn the latest fashions ... as both the shops and the contents of the windows in London are now quite on a level with anything to be seen in Nice or Paris.'[2]

FASHIONABLE INTELLIGENCE:
HEATHER FIRBANK'S FASHION ARCHIVE

The historical value of Heather's surviving wardrobe of garments and accessories is amplified by her collection of hundreds of bills and fashion cuttings from magazines and newspapers. These provide a unique source of evidence about the consumption of high fashion in London, particularly from 1908 until 1914, with sporadic pockets of information continuing to 1918. In 1964, the journalist Alison Adburgham illustrated some bills and documents from the Heather Firbank Collection for her still-standard book on the history of fashion retailing, *Shops and Shopping 1800–1914: Where and in What Manner the Well-dressed Englishwoman Bought Her Clothes*. Madeleine Ginsburg, the curator of the 1960 exhibition *A Lady of Fashion* [see **4**], had already foregrounded

110 Tailored jacket (detail of plate 32)
JACKET V&A: CIRC.646-1964
BLOUSE V&A: T.59-1960

Shopping with Heather Firbank

1   Reville & Rossiter *Court Dressmakers, 15 & 16 Hanover Square*

2   Hook, Knowles & Co. *Ladies' Boot and Shoe Manufacturer, 65 & 66 New Bond Street*

3   Maison Lewis *Modes, 152 Regent Street*

4   Lucile Ltd *Court Dressmakers, 23 Hanover Square*

5   The Irish Linen Stores *112 New Bond Street*

6   Alan McAfee Ltd *Boot and Shoe Manufacturer, 66 & 68 Duke Street*

7   Mascotte *Court Dressmaker, 89 Park Street, Park Lane (1907–13), and 12 & 13 Berkeley Street, Berkeley Square (1913–17)*

8   Pickett *Court Dressmaker, 20 Savile Row*

9   Frederick Bosworth *Ladies' Tailor & Court Dressmaker, 9 New Burlington Street*

10   Redfern *Ladies' Tailor, Court Dressmaker & Furrier, 26 & 27 Conduit Street, and 27 New Bond Street*

11   Scott Adie *Royal Cloak Maker and Royal Scotch Warehouse, 115 Regent Street*

12   Augustus Bide *Glove Manufacturer, 158A New Bond Street*

13   The Grafton Fur Company Ltd *164 New Bond Street*

14   Russell & Allen *Court Dressmakers and Milliners, 17–19 Old Bond Street*

15   J. Woodrow & Sons Ltd *Hat Manufacturers, 46 Piccadilly*

16   Cooper & Machinka *Court Dressmakers, 36 Dover Street*

17   Kate Reily Ltd *Court Dressmaker and Milliner, 10–12 Dover Street*

18   Floris *Perfumer, Comb and Brushmaker, 89 Jermyn Street*

19   11 Hill Street *Firbank residence to 1909*

20   33 Curzon Street *Firbank residence 1909–14*

21   Albert Minty *Coiffeur, Fleuriste, Parfumeur: Hairdressing Department, Hyde Park Hotel, Albert Gate*

22   Woolland Brothers *95–107 Knightsbridge*

23   Richard Sands & Co. *Court Glovers, Hosiers, Lacemen and Ladies Outfitters 188A & 189A Sloane Street*

24   Charles Lee *Court Dressmakers, 26–29 Sloane Street (1906–10)*

25   44 Sloane Street *Firbank residence 1914–19*

26   Mesdames Devalois & Rocher *Corsetières de Paris, 59 Beauchamp Place*

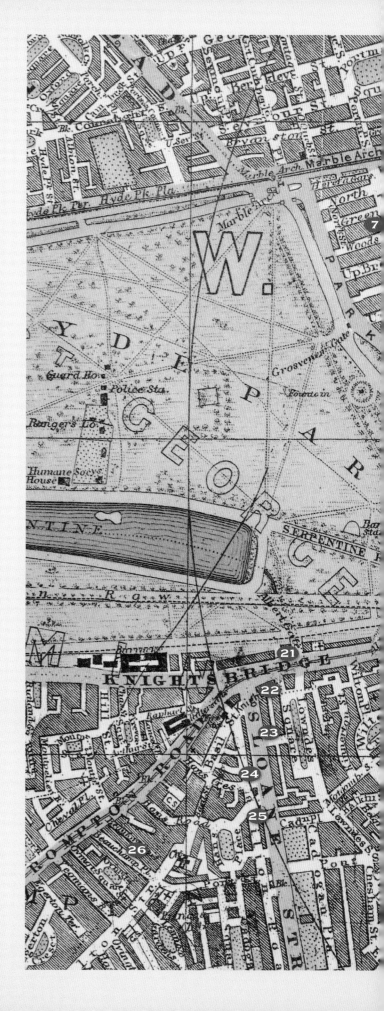

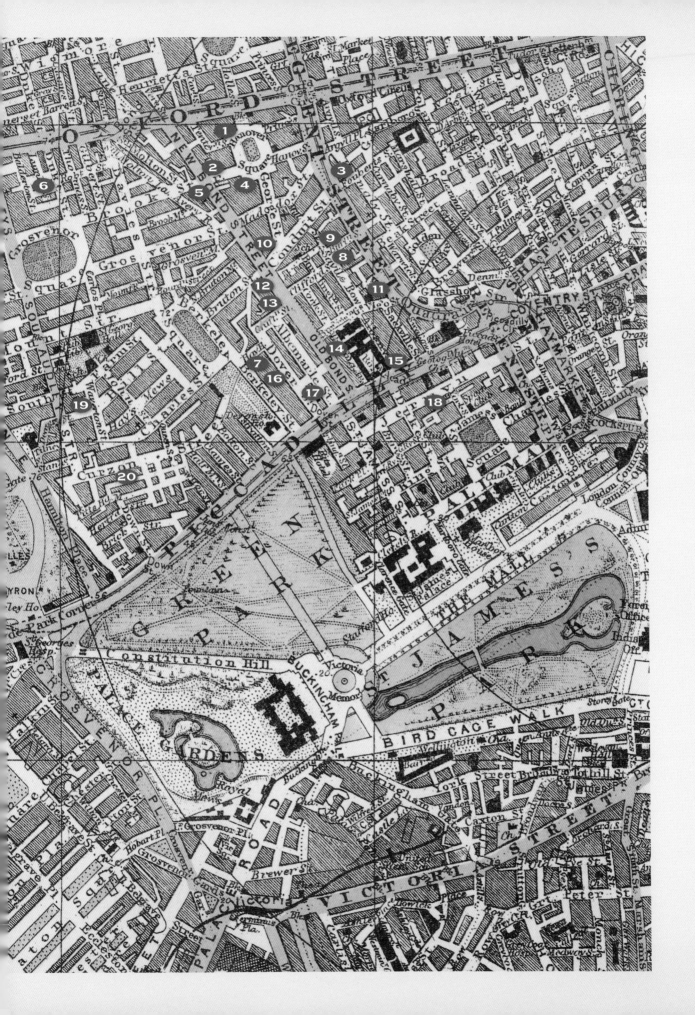

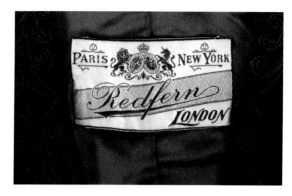

the importance of the bills and documents – literally, by covering the faces of the mannequins with pasted-on copies. She was also able to contact surviving family members and employees of the 25 firms represented in these documents and began to put the collection in a business context.

More recently Cassie Davies-Strodder's work has instigated renewed research into the department stores and dressmakers represented in the Heather Firbank Collection and archive of papers. A few of the firms lingered on into the late twentieth century, such as the shoemakers Alan McAfee, who survived until 1989. The department stores Debenhams and Peter Robinson (which became part of the Burton Group) still operate in the transformed retailing environment of the twenty-first century. However, most of the dressmaking firms used by Heather, such as Redfern and Kate Reily, despite once being internationally renowned, were out of business by the end of the Second World War. The Heather Firbank archive enables us to explore the forgotten world of Edwardian dressmakers revealed in the embroidered labels in the linings of Heather's clothes, printed at the head of her bills and described in the fashion articles she collected [111, 112].

The collection includes a few complete copies of *Les Modes*, the most exclusive Paris fashion magazine of the pre-war period, some copies of *Chiffons*, a French magazine produced just after the war, and many pages from *The Queen*, Britain's leading weekly women's magazine [113]. Single copies of other magazines, such as the *New Album of Modes: The Fashion Authority* from July 1907, indicate the wide range of material available to Heather and her contemporaries. The archive is dominated, however, by the 'For and About Women' pages from the *Evening Standard and St James's Gazette*, which Heather received at 33 Curzon Street and, from 1914, at 44 Sloane Street. She collected these pages assiduously from 1908 to 1914 and seems to have focused on the fashion drawings by Bessie Ascough. (Bessie Ascough's drawings were a great source of inspiration

to Cecil Beaton as a young boy.[3]) A detailed commentary for the fashion drawings is provided by an anonymous author, and the surrounding advertisements and editorial about subjects such as cleaning lace, children's clothes, suggested daily menus and shopping in London's regular sales provide a wealth of information about lifestyles and the wider world of fashion retailing, as well as further evidence of the work produced by the dressmakers who supplied Heather's distinctive dresses, tailoring and accessories [114].

Bessie Ascough trained in figure drawing at the art school in Bedford Park, Chiswick, the west London suburb built in the 'Aesthetic' style. Her fashion drawings for the *Evening Standard and St James's Gazette* and the *Daily Mail* were syndicated in other newspapers across the English-speaking world, in the United States and in Australia, and her distinctive style was of the moment – she was selected to provide illustrations for publicity for the opening of Selfridges in 1909. Her signature sometimes led to confusion and she was often credited as the designer of the fashions in her drawings, but her career developed into fashion journalism rather than design. Certainly by 1914 she was supplying written fashion advice and news on the latest fashions from Paris to the *New York Tribune*.[4] Heather's collection of 'For and About Women' pages reflects the demand for regular information about fashion by the readers of London's evening newspaper. Priced at a penny, it reached a large number of the

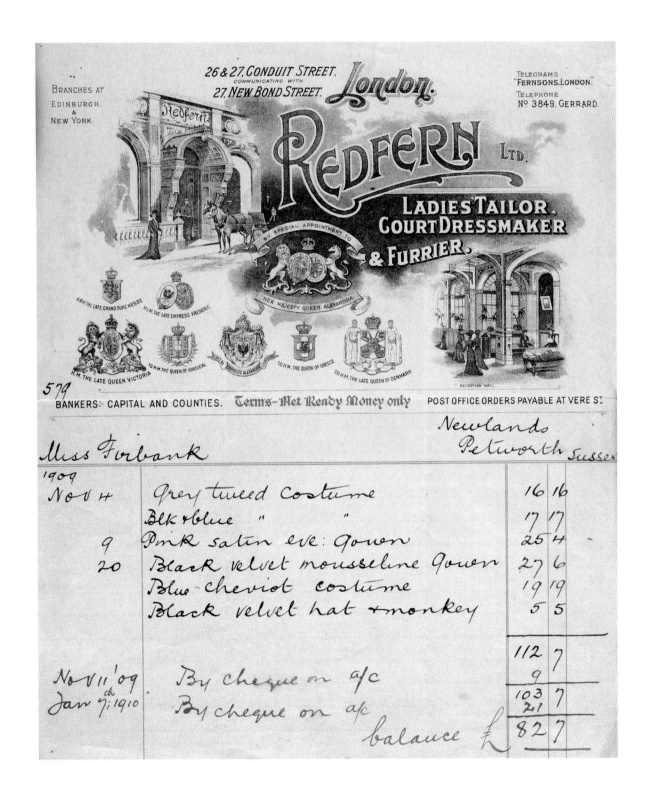

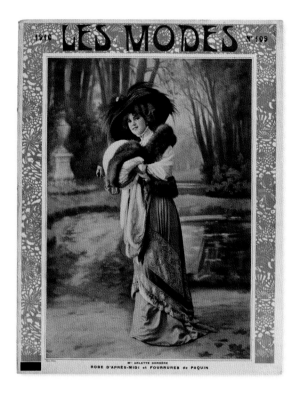

113 'Robe d'après-midi et fourrures de Paquin', *Les Modes*, January 1910

V&A: HEATHER FIRBANK ARCHIVE

114 Full-page spread showing dress by Reville & Rossiter, illustrated by Bessie Ascough, *Evening Standard and St James's Gazette*, London, 7 May 1910, the day after Edward VII's death

V&A: HEATHER FIRBANK ARCHIVE

clothes. The unique combination in the West End of royal and aristocratic residences, public parks and squares, theatres, clubs and shops, gave the 'golden rectangle' bordered by Piccadilly, Regent Street, Oxford Street and Park Lane an unrivalled position as the hub of the British Empire's international power, wealth and pleasure.[5] The flourishing retail economy and the personal activity of shopping were obvious demonstrations of confidence in London as the most developed city in the world.

In 1908, there were over 1,700 dressmakers listed in the London Post Office directory and 5 per cent were described as 'court' dressmakers. There were also many milliners, which by this date had become the term used purely for shops retailing hats. (Until the second half of the nineteenth century the term 'milliners' was used for the proprietors of establishments creating and selling entire ensembles – dresses and accessories. It was not until after the First World War that some London dressmakers gave themselves the title 'couturier' or 'couturière', borrowed from the French fashion houses.) Many court dressmakers could be found to the north of Oxford Street, clustered around Manchester Square and Wigmore Street, and to the south-west in Belgravia, particularly around Sloane Street and the department stores of Knightsbridge, but most were concentrated in the streets and squares of Mayfair and on Bond Street, which runs north from Piccadilly to Oxford Street. This had become a fashionable shopping street in the mid-eighteenth century, and 150 years later there were many different trades existing side by side, with shops catering for men at the southern end and the newer shops for women's clothes, shoes and gloves in New Bond Street to the north [115].

A flavour of the reserved atmosphere of this exclusive thoroughfare is given by Virginia Woolf's description in *Mrs Dalloway* (1925) of the mixed trades still operating there after the war. Clarissa Dalloway goes shopping for flowers there one morning: 'Bond Street fascinated her; Bond Street early in the morning in the season; its flags flying; its shops; no splash;

city's female population, although only a small proportion of them would have been in a position to purchase clothes from the dressmakers' shops featured in the articles.

THE PRE-WAR COURT DRESSMAKING WORLD
London's clothing industry encompassed a huge range of establishments catering for the needs of customers at every level of society. The nineteenth century had seen the growth of an army of unregulated and unprotected workers, producing cheap ready-made garments and accessories in unhealthy sweatshops – effectively small factories without sanitation, ventilation or light, particularly in London's East End. Across the city, there were many thousands of outworkers making shirts or accessories as piecework in their homes, while many bespoke clothes were made by private dressmakers. Shops and wholesalers were still based in the area around St Paul's Cathedral, London's original fashion centre, but most luxury shops, as today, were located in the streets surrounding Bond Street. These shops were converted from residential homes built in the eighteenth century, with grand showrooms on the ground floor and fitting rooms above, with workrooms and sometimes accommodation for staff on the upper floors. The department stores of nearby Oxford Street and Regent Street catered additionally for a wider range of social groups, providing ready-made and made-to-measure

FOR AND ABOUT WOMEN

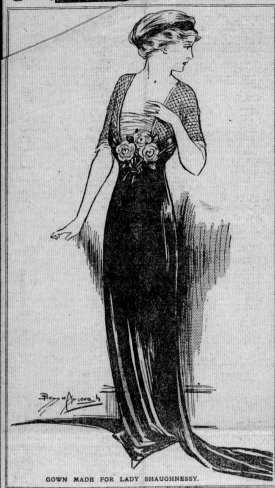

GOWN MADE FOR LADY SHAUGHNESSY.

TO-DAY'S FASHION.

Charming Black Velvet Gown Made for Lady Shaughnessy.

LATTICE WORK OF ALUMINIUM CHAINS AND DIAMONDS.

The va et vient between Canada and England has surely never been so marked as it has this year.

The link which binds the land of snows with the Old Country seems of late to have been growing stronger than ever, and the trip to England is accounted in these times as an everyday matter. On the other hand we, in our turn, find infinite possibilities for enjoyment in even a short holiday spent in Canada, and the return visits to friends on one side and the other have become almost the ordinary events of existence. The couturieres, too, have been almost as busy in carrying out the orders of visitors from Canada as they have with their clients on this side, and the result has been a bevy of lovely toilettes for all occasions.

CLUSTER OF GARDENIAS.

A notable example is the beautiful gown made for Lady Shaughnessy, wife of Sir Thomas Shaughnessy, President of the Canadian Pacific Railway Company. This, which is sketched on this page, and which has been designed and made by Messrs. Reville and Rossiter, 15, Hanover-square, W., is carried out in black velvet, falling in rich sculptured folds to the feet.

The gown is exquisitely moulded over the hips and softly wrinkled round the waist, the folds in front being caught into a big oval buckle formed of a twisted roll of black velvet through which is thrust two or three snow-white gardenias, their waxen petals flanked by a few dark glossy leaves.

PALE FLESH PINK TULLE.

Above the soft mat black of the velvet is the corsage composed of a lattice work of fine aluminium chains crossed and recrossed in lattice work fashion, and studded with a large mock diamond at each intersecting point, which glitters like blue fire with every movement of the wearer. The chain-work is mounted over the palest flesh pink tulle, the colour being so faint as to suggest scarcely more than the reflection of a sunset cloud on a bank of snow. The sleeves, which are of elbow length, are made all in one with the corsage, and are mounted over the palest flesh pink chiffon to match the gown, a fold of pink velvet edging them at the hem.

In front where the "chain armour" of aluminium falls away on either side the corsage is filled in with soft folds of pink chiffon arranged horizontally, this arrangement softening the effect and giving distinction to the scheme.

TO-MORROW'S MENUS AND PLAT DU JOUR.

LUNCH.
Curried eggs and fonds d'artichauts.
Roast chicken.
Ham creams. Cold galantine of veal aux pistaches.
Chocolate soufflé.

DINNER.
Oxtail soup.
Lobster mayonnaise aux fines herbes.
Blanquette of veal en casserole.
Aspic of quails. Salad.
Strawberry pineapple. Lemon custards.

NOVELTIES IN BREAD.

Never, surely, in the history of baking has the staff of life been prepared in so many attractive forms. This enterprise on the part of bakers began a few years ago with the introduction of currant bread—or, rather, its re-introduction, for currant bread was popular a generation ago—and so immediate and pronounced was the success of this article, that ever since the artists in dough have been exercising their ingenuity to devise new dainties. There is nothing tastier or more wholesome than currant bread in any form. When cut very thin and spread with fresh butter, it is delicious, either for afternoon tea or as a snack between meals, and it has the added advantage of being highly nutritious.

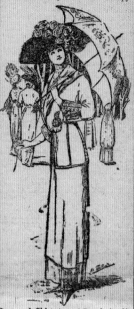
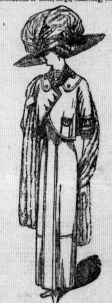
OUR NATIONAL LOSS.

Every Woman's Tribute to King Edward VII.

We are all mourners together to-day.

In the presence of the Angel of Death every other consideration seems to be swept away. The whole nation has been watching, so to speak, at the King's deathbed, and the vigil is over. The King is dead.

It is only left for us now to realise the loss which is paralysing us for the moment.

Apart from the qualities of a great leader, a far-seeing and wise director, it was the more intimate qualities of the King's kingliness which most appealed to women. The exquisite tact—a Royal inheritance from a Royal mother—the tact which sprang partly from the innate geniality and sweetness of the King's disposition, partly from his great knowledge of human nature, and partly from that indefinable quality, that mysterious aura which is acknowledged without being seen, and which proclaims a man a gentleman, whether he is born in a hovel or a palace.

Women were very proud of the King's tact. The hero worship which is buried deep down in every woman's heart found much to admire in the smile which smoothed away difficulties, as if by magic, the right word spoken at the right moment, and the graceful and kingly action which was so powerful to bring order and good fellowship out of chaos.

But if the King's tact roused our enthusiasm, we were still prouder of the charm of manner which was a proverb with all those who knew Edward VII. We boasted of the quality of personal magnetism which won him hosts of devoted friends in every continent, and will hallow his memory to the generations of English subjects who will come after us. The quality which makes Royalists wherever Royalty goes, which can hold the affections of an Empire in the hollow of its hand, is indeed a kingly gift. It was such a quality which brought freedom to Cœur de Lion in the old days through the devotion of a little page; which won Crecy and Agincourt, and inspired the pen of Spenser, and kept a devoted Court round Mary Queen of Scots in the last days of her long captivity. It is the quality which created heroes and strategists wherever the wandering of Charles Stuart led him, and which has caused every sword to spring from its scabbard in defence of its idol whenever that quality has existed in leader or sovereign.

And above all these we ranked his rôle as peacemaker. No words are needed to describe what such a quality means to women in general, how deep a feeling of gratitude and love it rouses in our hearts.

And in the midst of our personal grief for the loss of our King, in the midst of our conning over the gracious gifts which have endeared him to his subjects in every corner of the world, our hearts are aching for the Royal lady on whom the heaviest burden of sorrow has fallen to-day, and the prayer in every woman's heart will be, "God comfort the Queen."

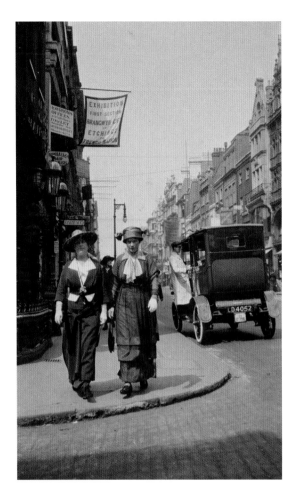

and family mourning as specialities. The company remained in business for 83 years, closing in 1941. In newspaper reports in the 1890s and early 1900s, Russell & Allen are often credited with supplying the court dresses for debutantes and attendees at Queen Victoria's drawing rooms.[7] Other residential streets off Piccadilly, such as Dover Street, also became important retail thoroughfares as the address of elite dressmakers such as Kate Reily and the French couturière Paquin, who opened a shop there in 1896.

FAVOURITE COUTURIERS

None of Heather's diaries survive, but those published by other society women show that they all had their preferred couturiers and milliners, who played a central role in producing the personal style of their clients – their public personas. Cynthia Asquith's favourite milliner when a debutante was Maison St Louis, where Miss Louise Piers plied her art, 'creating (in this connection the word is fully justified) the lovely original hats for which she was famed ... My favourite dressmaker was Madame Marte, who specialised in the sheening ball gowns we called our "fish-dresses" – lovely skin tight sheaths of gold, silver or sea-coloured tissue.' Women would also engage the services of private dressmakers to make less special garments – the 'little woman' 'who had no models but only paper patterns', though often these were 'not right'.[8] The personal maids (like Heather's maid, Adelaide Hallett) of aristocratic and upper-class women were also often skilled dressmakers who would help to make clothes for their employer and her daughters. Lady Angela Forbes, who married in 1896, remembered that in her debutante years she

had a lovely white frock made by Mrs Mason. She was 'it' in the dressmaker line; all her models came direct from Jean Worth, and anyone who had any pretension to dressing well in those days bought their frocks from her. She was a most perfect old lady and might have been a duchess instead of a dressmaker. Her prices were supposed to be exorbitant.[9]

no glitter; one roll of tweed in the shop where her father had bought his suits for fifty years; a few pearls; salmon on an iceblock.'[6]

Court dressmakers based on Bond Street, such as Madame Hayward (who was very well known at the time but is not represented in Heather's wardrobe or bills), Russell & Allen and their many competitors, produced or retailed the entire range of garments required by fashionable women for different functions and times of day, from fur coats to millinery, lingerie and corsetry. Russell & Allen (who supplied Heather with striking black woollen city walking coats, satin tea coats and various accessories, including veiling and handbags) evolved out of a traditional textile retail business and the company first appears in the Post Office directories in 1858 as 'Silk Mercers and Lacemen' at 18 Old Bond Street [116–120]. Fifty years later the company had expanded into the neighbouring houses on each side and, despite their simple billhead design listing their trade as 'Court dressmakers and Milliners', they also offered themselves as 'Furriers, mantlemakers, India and colonial outfitters and hosiers' and included tea gowns

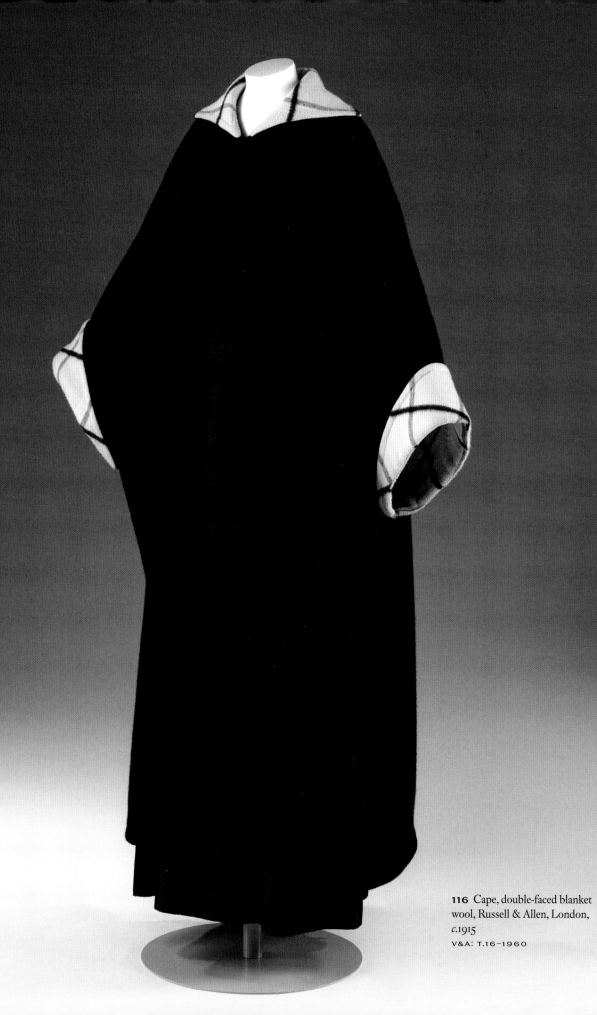

116 Cape, double-faced blanket
wool, Russell & Allen, London,
*c.*1915
V&A: T.16-1960

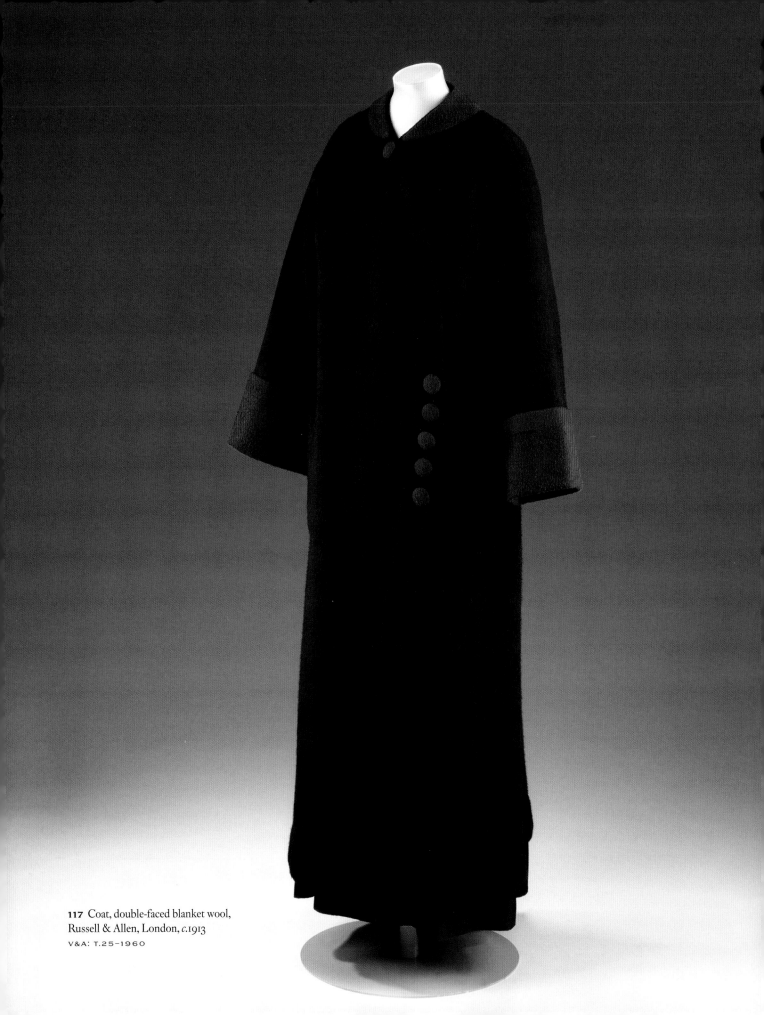

117 Coat, double-faced blanket wool,
Russell & Allen, London, *c.*1913

V&A: T.25-1960

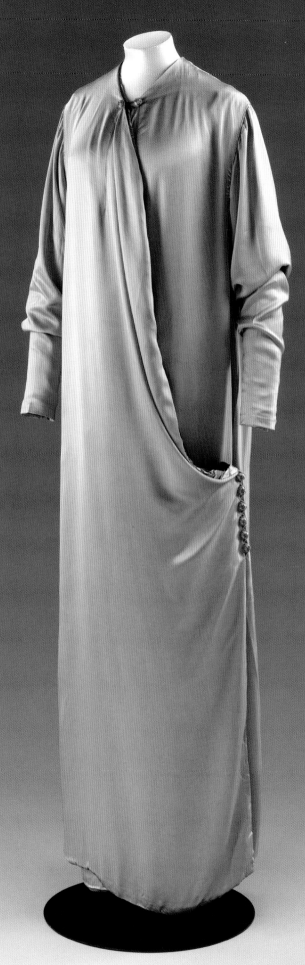

118 Tea coat, silk satin, Russell & Allen,
London, *c.*1915
V&A: T.46–1960

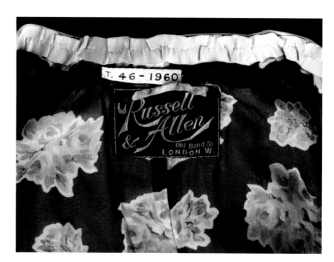

When the formidable Mrs Mason's shop at 4 New Burlington Street closed in 1902, the same address became the showroom and workrooms for Worth (London). The prices at Worth were legendary: a letter in a private collection of 1910 shows that an evening dress trimmed with jet and 'white diamonds' was priced at 950 francs (approximately £37 10s).[10] British women from the wealthiest and most aristocratic backgrounds went to the showrooms of Parisian couturiers to organize their wardrobes for the London season. Meanwhile, most London court dressmakers deliberately emulated Paris fashions, buying original models from Paris couturiers which they were then allowed to copy and adapt for their London clients. Some, however, such as Mrs Nettleship of Wigmore Street, were known to be more artistic and created more original designs.

'WHERE FASHION FASCINATES': KATE REILY OF DOVER STREET

Established Victorian court dressmakers such as Mrs Mason, Madame Hayward and Kate Reily (where Heather was a customer) marketed themselves on their ability to provide a modified form of fashions from Paris suited to British women and visitors to London from North America and the colonies. Kate Reily was one of a few English dressmakers who did not adopt a French-sounding name. Famous at the time, she has become one of the most elusive dressmakers of the nineteenth and early twentieth centuries, perhaps because so much of her work, like that of many other once well-known London dressmakers, has perished.[11] Dresses made in the 1890s, 1900s and 1910s were often composed of delicate layers of pale chiffon and silk, built on a foundation of tin-weighted silk, and decorated with appliquéd panels or beads, and these elaborate constructions have fallen into shreds because the metallic salts used to add weight have corroded the fragile textile.

Only a single dress by Kate Reily survives in the Heather Firbank Collection. Dating from about

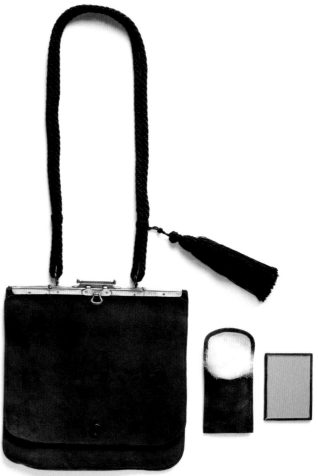

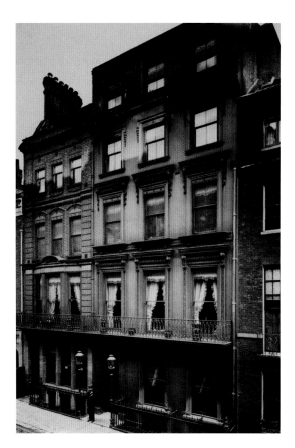

121 Kate Reily, 11 & 12 Dover Street, London,
19 November 1888
ENGLISH HERITAGE

1909, it is made of a fine ribbed silk, with a high-waisted bodice trimmed with chemical lace, with a chiffon over-bodice, frilled 'Romney' collar (named after the eighteenth-century portrait painter) and elbow-length sleeves. The dress is now too fragile to safely display on a mannequin and has been photographed flat [122, 123]. It is similar to the one worn by Heather in the portrait of her in a surviving hat by Woolland Brothers [see 1]. She also bought a 'pink Tagal (straw) hat with cotton scarf and rose' for £4 14s 6d, invoiced on 12 June 1908, but this no longer exists. Very few other Kate Reily dresses survive in public museum collections,[12] although the dressmaker's work appears quite frequently in reports of fashionable weddings in newspapers, including the *New York Times*.[13] The French couturière Vionnet is also thought to have worked in her establishment as a young woman in the 1890s.[14]

Kate Reily was the professional name of Harriet Reily, who was born in 1846, at which time her father was a house agent living in Bloomsbury. 'Kate Reily' is first listed in the Post Office directory in 1878 as a milliner at 100 Mount Street, Berkeley Square, although by the census in 1881 she had married Major Arthur Griffiths, at that time an Inspector of Prisons at Wormwood Scrubs.[15] Her business moved to 11 Dover Street, where it expanded, occupying numbers 10 and 12 by 1900, and becoming a limited company in 1902 [121].

A few streets west of Bond Street, Dover Street was the location of private hotels, elite dressmakers and luxurious clubs (such as the Hogarth Club, at 36 until 1898, and Heather's club, the Ladies' Imperial Club, at 17), and the street had become 'the first great shopping rendezvous of the season' by 1909.[16] Kate Reily's business had expanded in the 1880s, as demonstrated by advertisements in provincial newspapers such as the *Yorkshire Post* and the *Leeds Mercury* for staff, including 'improvers' (girls who had completed a basic apprenticeship), 'good assistant skirt hands' and 'good low bodice-trimmers'. Similar advertisements continue into the 1890s, stressing the need for

staff to be 'tall and have a good figure' for 'trying on', indicating that sewing hands effectively also worked as models.[17] Other notices in the press reveal that one key element of her business strategy was the flexibility to accommodate both elaborate toilettes and simple and inexpensive costumes, while 'evincing the same care and excellent taste'.[18]

Kate Reily also promoted herself by association with illustrious clients, such as Queen Victoria's granddaughter Princess Helena of Schleswig-Holstein, the Duchess of Manchester, and several wealthy American women, including members of the Kellogg and Vanderbilt families. By 1887 she was sending 'a representative to New York with a number of her newest fashions'[19] and a few years later she had established branches of her business in New York and Chicago, although the American operation ended in 1894, when her stock was purchased by Ehrich Brothers of New York and many 'magnificent costumes' were sold off at a fraction of the original price.[20] This conclusion of Kate Reily's American operation may have been connected with an earlier accusation from an employee, a Mrs E.C. Wade, that the company regularly sent young dressmakers to New York with 'large quantities of wraps and Parisian robes' in their baggage without paying import duties and thus violating customs

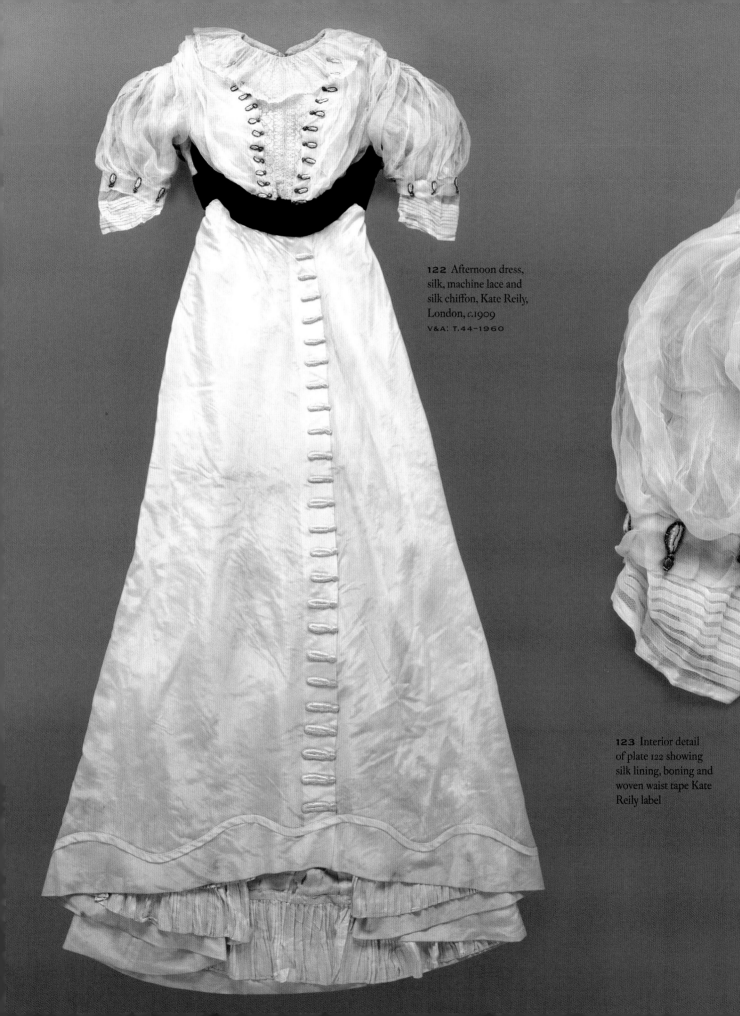

122 Afternoon dress, silk, machine lace and silk chiffon, Kate Reily, London, *c.*1909
V&A: T.44-1960

123 Interior detail of plate 122 showing silk lining, boning and woven waist tape Kate Reily label

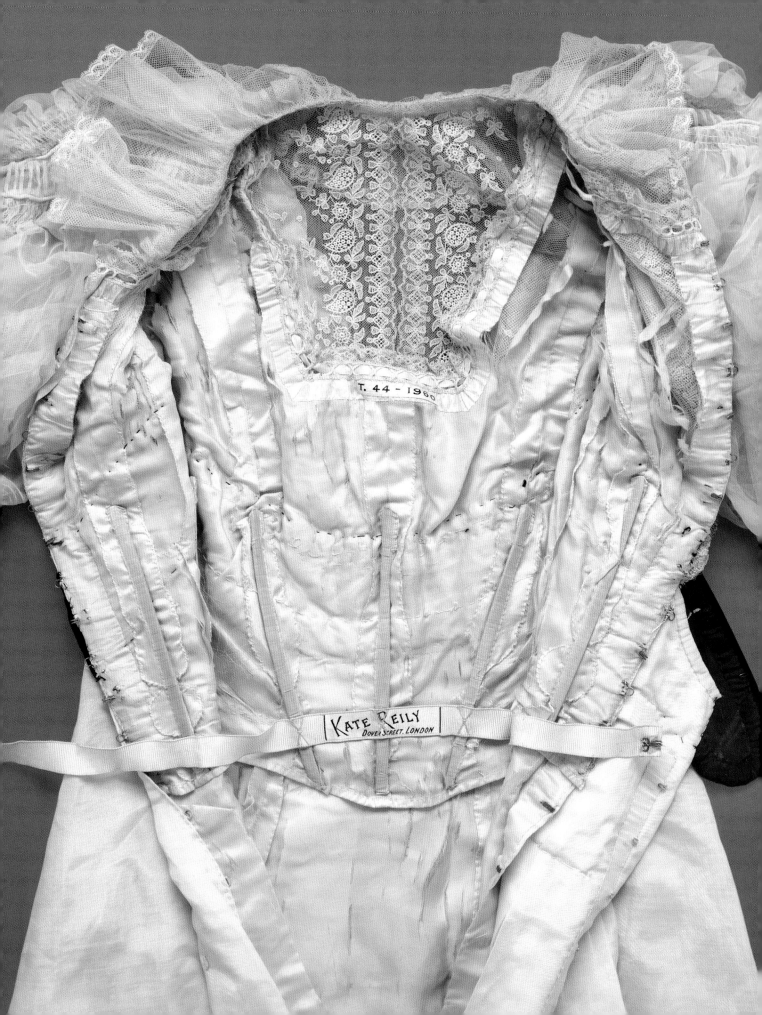

T. 44 - 1960

KATE REILY
DOVER STREET, LONDON

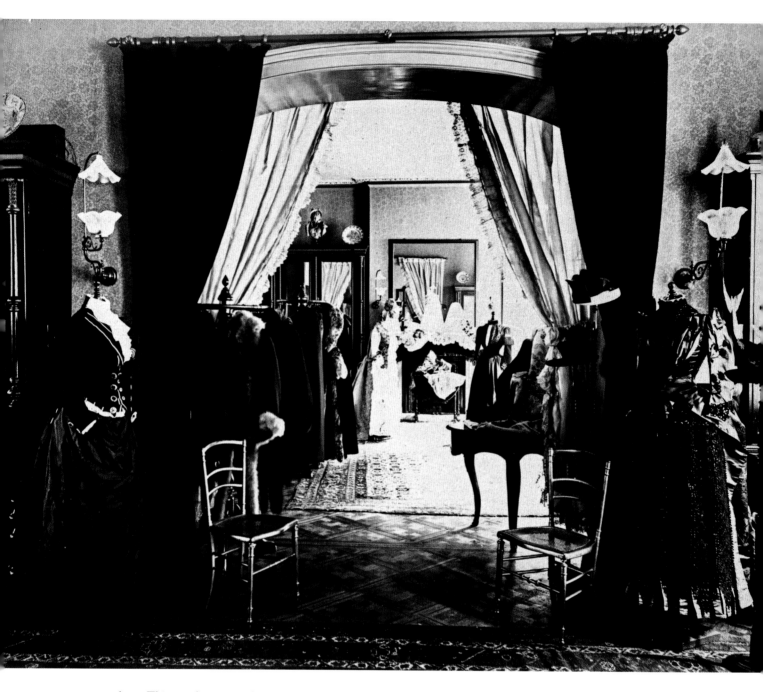

laws. This revelation resulted in a US Government investigation.[21]

A rare photograph gives us a glimpse of Kate Reily's London showroom in 1888, the year Heather was born [124]. Worth had established the importance of a suitably lavish setting for selling fashion, and the decorative style, typical of 'high' Victorian domestic interiors, is suitably welcoming, with curtains, parquet flooring and machine-woven rugs, and with ceramics providing interesting focal points. Dresses are shown mounted on dressmaking bust forms, with free-standing racks for hanging mantles and

coats. This view contrasts with Lady Duff-Gordon's assertion that, in the 1890s, dressmakers' clients were 'received into the uncompromising atmosphere of a shop, with hard chairs, a few unbecoming mirrors and a door, which opened on to a little fitting room'.[22]

Kate Reily's business continued for a further 26 years, but it was at its most successful in the period just before and after 1900. She featured frequently in magazines: for example, in the *Gentlewoman* of 2 March 1901, she – an imposing presence aged 56 – is depicted as the personification of 'Dame Fashion', charming the writer of an article entitled 'Where

Fashion Fascinates' in one of her designs for mourning dress (for the death of Queen Victoria). This is described as a 'lovely black day-frock of crêpe de chine, tucked and appliquéd with medallions of black Chantilly lace, transparent to reveal the white under-slip', hinting at the great potential for suggestive layering of delicate laces and fabrics, particularly in mourning. However, advertising in the early 1900s in traditional magazines such as *Country Life* suggests that, inevitably, Kate Reily's clients were ageing.[23]

Kate Reily died childless in 1908, at the age of 62, although her shop continued to trade on a reduced scale from 11 and 12 Dover Street. Clearly emulating the successful house style of Lucile, the managers refurbished the shop in 1909 in an attempt to retain and attract customers, creating a series of new fitting rooms furnished in an 'artistic fashion ... [carrying] more the impression of "my Lady's Boudoir" than a fashionable couturieres salon', as the *Observer's* 'Seen at the Shops' columnist reported.[24] The showroom was decorated with a laurel-leaf patterned wallpaper and a chintz of 'bold hollyhock design in natural colourings'. Despite this, Kate Reily was not able to compete with the new generation of court dress-makers and the business finally went into voluntary receivership in 1914, after trading for 36 years. The entire stock was sold in the 'outstanding shopping event of the Autumn' at Barkers department store on Kensington High Street, on 23 November of that year. An advertisement listed the great range of 'superb silks', costumes, furs, millinery, ties and muffs sold at less than a third of their previous value.

Perhaps Kate Reily's most outstanding achievement was to be internationally known as a London dressmaker, with branches in New York and Chicago, like the London firm Redfern – and 20 years before Lucile followed this lead. Further research may reveal other enterprising nineteenth-century transatlantic businesswomen like her.[25]

EDWARDIAN DRESSMAKERS: PICKETT, REVILLE & ROSSITER, MASCOTTE AND MACHINKA

Heather Firbank patronized other now unknown Edwardian dressmakers, including a Mrs Pickett, who ran her business at 20 Savile Row from 1892 to 1922. From 1905, she was listed in Post Office directories as a court costumier. Mrs Pickett's workroom staff made Heather's beautiful pale lilac silk afternoon dress of 1909 [**125**]. Two other very delicate early Edwardian styles by the same dressmaker survive at the Museum of London, but otherwise little is known about her, although a newspaper report of August 1890 shows that Mrs Pickett's husband was involved in the business, as he sued a customer's husband for unpaid bills.[26]

Among the younger dressmakers making a name for themselves, and also attracting Heather's custom, was the partnership of Reville & Rossiter of Hanover Square. Although no labelled garments survive in the Heather Firbank Collection, bills show that she was a regular customer of this recently established firm, at least in 1908 and 1909, as she was billed for an ivory satin evening gown costing 22 guineas on Christmas Eve 1908 and a pink satin evening gown costing 20 guineas in November 1909, while another evening gown of ivory satin, listed with a diamond headdress, a pearl headdress, a white linen coat and skirt, and a yellow linen coat skirt, was made for her in December of the same year [see **2**]. Heather's grand beaded ball gown of around 1909 is conceivably from Reville & Rossiter, as they were well known for their beautiful evening dresses [**126**].

The company was formed in 1905 by William Wallace Reville Terry (1870–1948), the mantle buyer at Jay's, a department store, and Sarah Rossiter, who was the tea gown buyer at the same shop.[27] Jay's opened on Regent Street in 1841 as a 'general mourning ware-house' and became a highly successful business. After only a few years, Reville & Rossiter had become two of the most celebrated names in Edwardian dress-making, receiving the royal warrant in 1910.

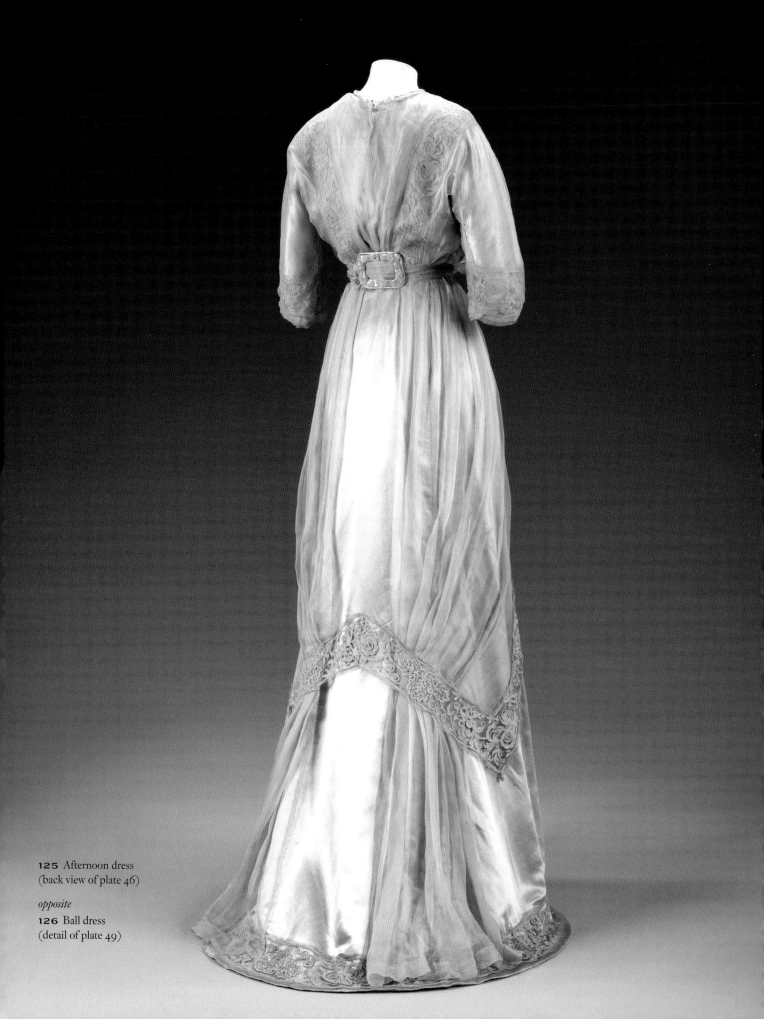

125 Afternoon dress
(back view of plate 46)

opposite

126 Ball dress
(detail of plate 49)

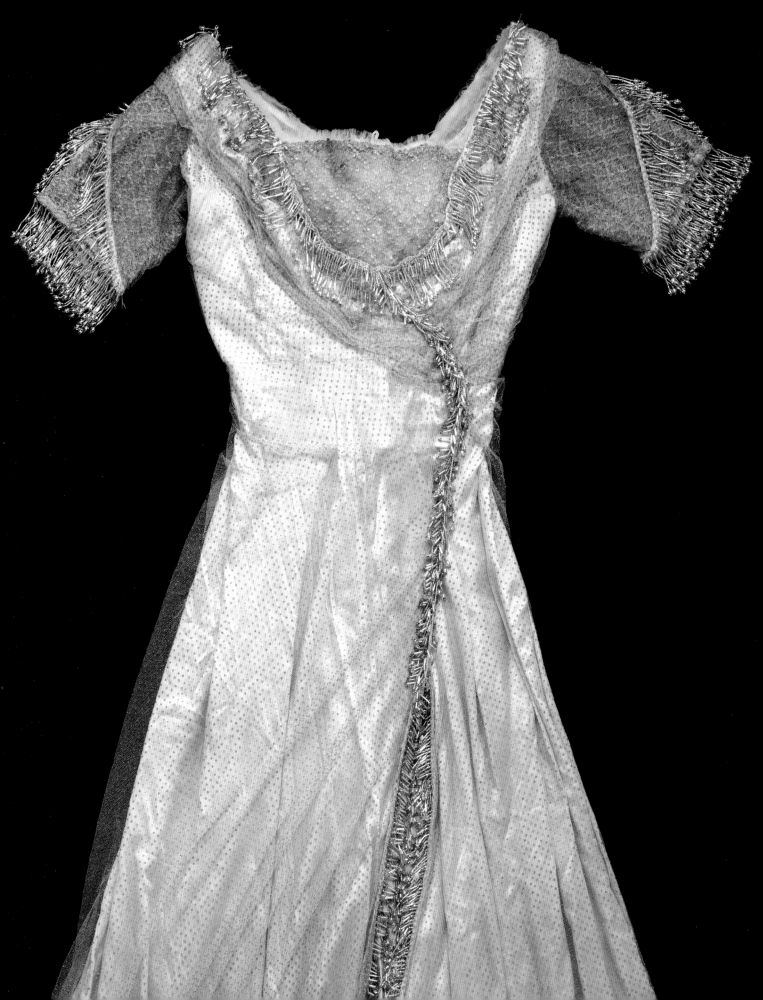

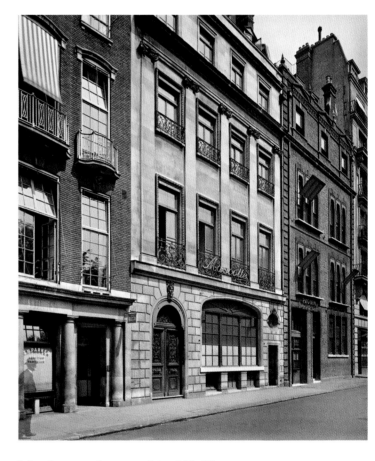

According to Charlotte Mortimer, who began her career at Reville & Rossiter, while at Jay's the partnership had built up 'the most distinguished, as well as the most profitable, clientele in London', and many of these prestigious customers would have brought their patronage to the new company. Interviewed in 1953, Mortimer describes how she 'shook like a jelly' when interviewed by Miss Rossiter for her first position as a model for the firm. Mortimer had two children and 'had never expected to earn her living'. But, as an accomplished horsewoman and a fencer, she had a good figure and she got the job. Initially she worked the long hours (from 9am until 7pm during the week and until 2pm on Saturday) as an apprentice for nothing, eventually earning 10 shillings a week. Apparently discipline was strict, even for the time, but perhaps because of this the company was successful, establishing a reputation for beautiful wedding and court dresses. Reville & Rossiter made many of Queen Mary's clothes, including her coronation gown in 1911. William Terry became the sole designer for the firm after 1912, although the company's name did not change until 1919, when it became Reville Ltd. The company went into voluntary liquidation in 1926, despite its growing international success, when William Terry left the company to set up independently. London couturier Victor Stiebel began his career there in the late 1920s, and the name of Reville remained at the heart of the London couture industry until after the Second World War, incorporating Worth (London) at 50 Grosvenor Street from 1936 until 1949. The Worth (London) house finally closed in 1970.[28]

The two court dressmaking companies most closely associated with Heather Firbank and represented so richly in her wardrobe are Redfern and Lucile, each long-associated with separate key developments in fashion, sporting and businesslike tailor-made costumes, and romantic, sensual tea gowns. The work of a third dressmaker, Mascotte, is very little known apart from the evidence of a few garments in the collections of the V&A and the Gallery of Costume in Manchester and two surviving bills. The garments at the V&A include two day dresses, an unusual purple tailored jacket and skirt, and a stunning black silk satin tea coat lined with palest lilac silk [**30, 129, 130, 133**].

Though portrayed in the 1960 *Lady of Fashion* exhibition as a woman of 'high' birth working in a trade, Madame Mascotte was in fact an example of the social mobility possible in this period. Madame Mascotte was the professional name of dressmaker Mrs Cyril Drummond. She was born Edith Belle Wilkins in Southampton in 1871, the daughter of a clerk working for the London and South-West Railway. In the 1891 census she is listed as a dressmaker living with her parents in the fashionable resort of Cowes, on the Isle of Wight, and it seems likely that

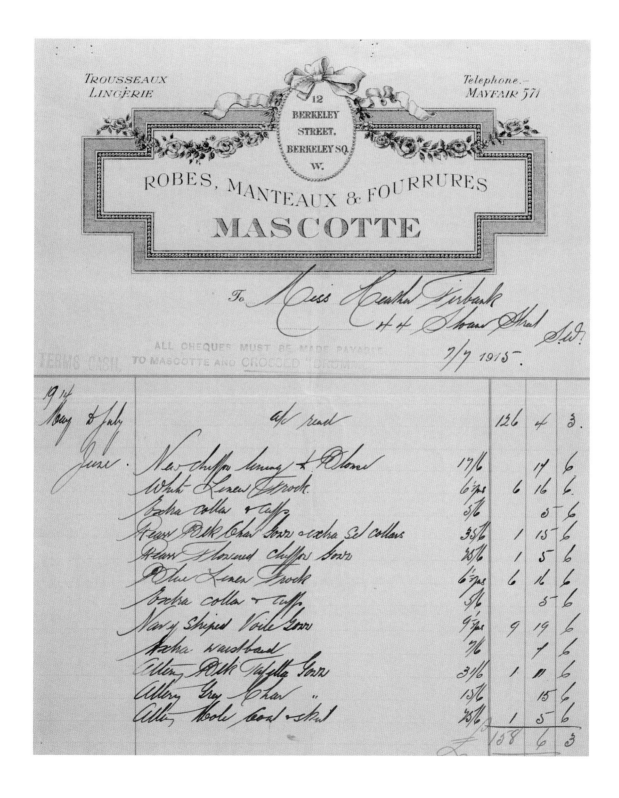

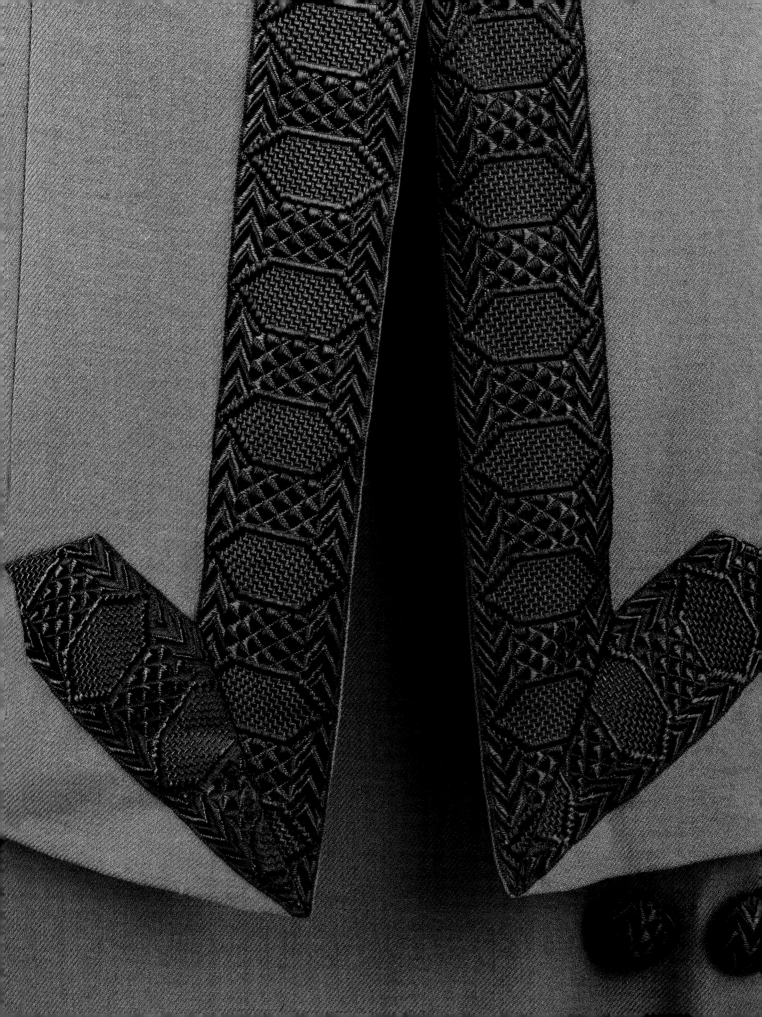

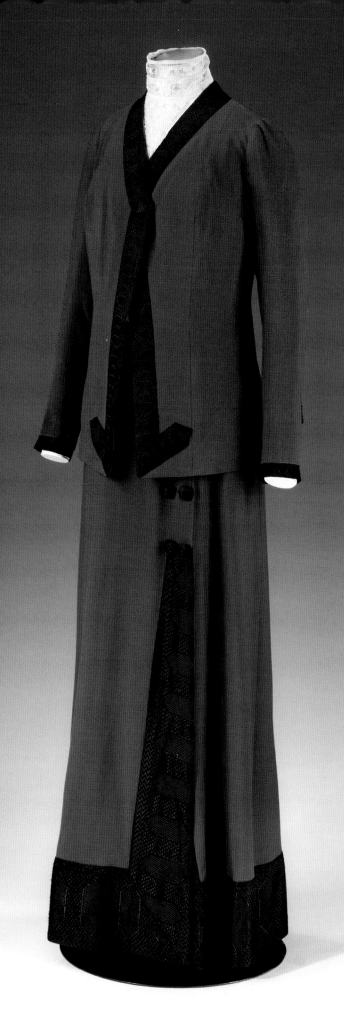

129 Tailored jacket and skirt, wool serge, trimmed with silk jacquard braid, Mascotte, London, *c.*1912

V&A: T.43&A-1960

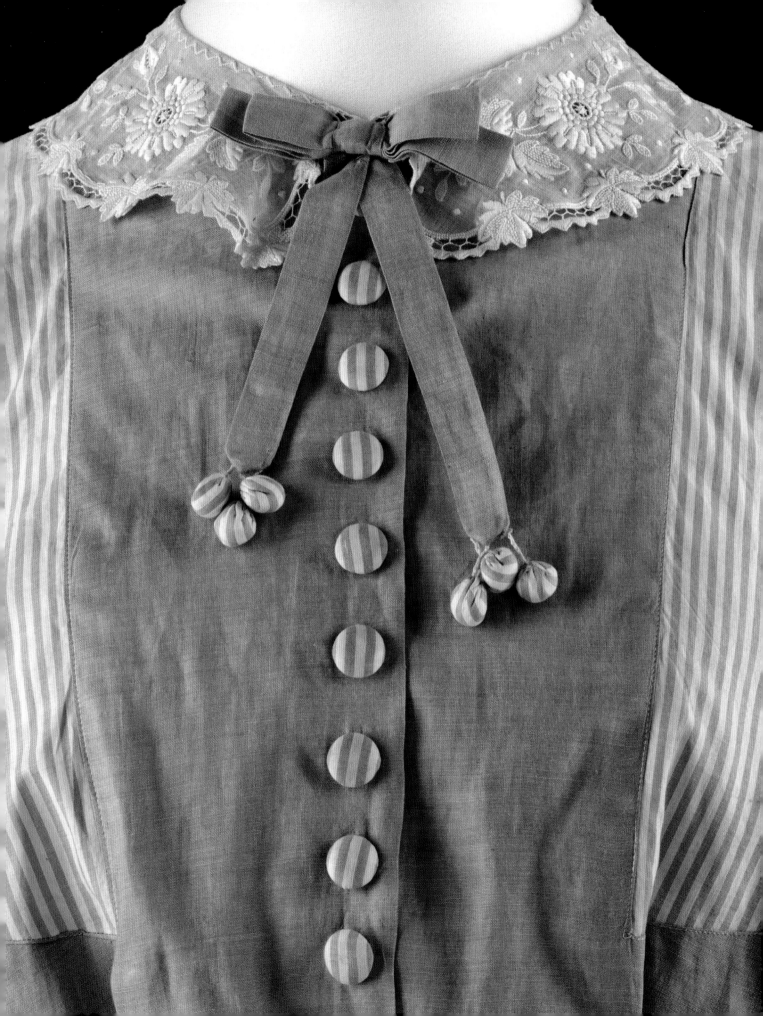

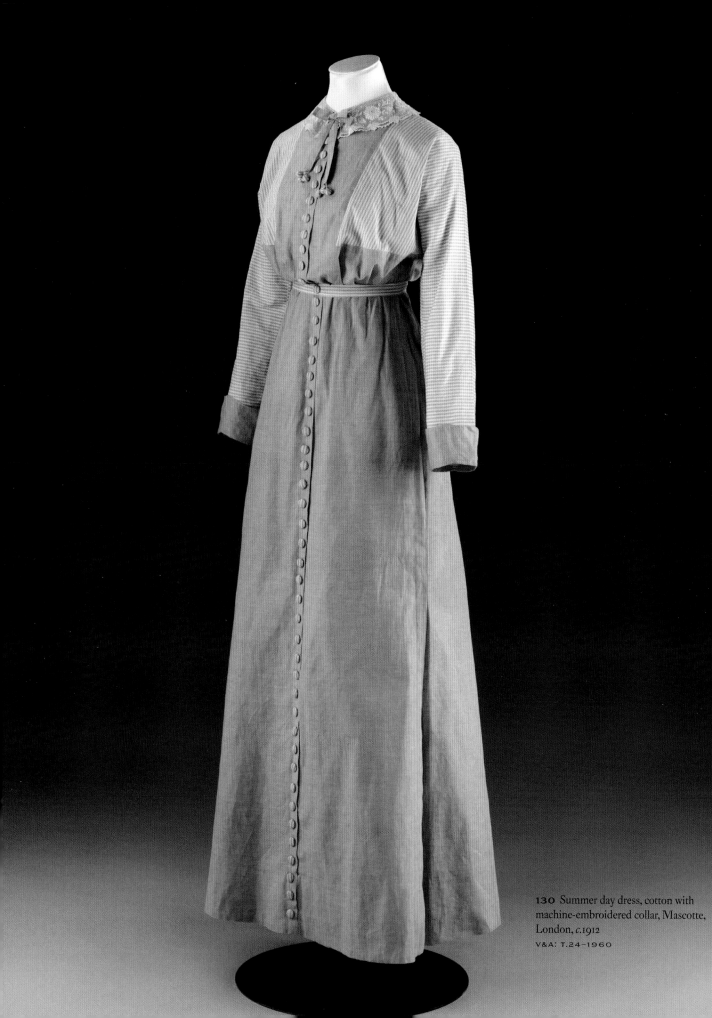

130 Summer day dress, cotton with
machine-embroidered collar, Mascotte,
London, *c.*1912
V&A: T.24–1960

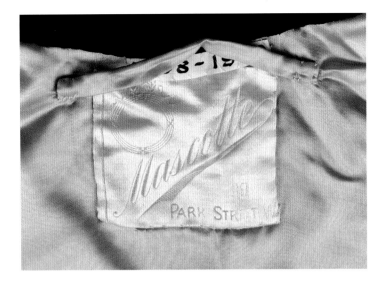

131 Detail of plate 133 showing silk satin Mascotte label

132 Rest gown by Mascotte, illustrated by Bessie Ascough, cutting from the *Evening Standard and St James's Gazette*, 25 March 1914
V&A: HEATHER FIRBANK ARCHIVE

133 Tea coat, silk satin with silk frogging fastening, lined with silk satin, Mascotte, London, *c.*1912
V&A: T.98–1960

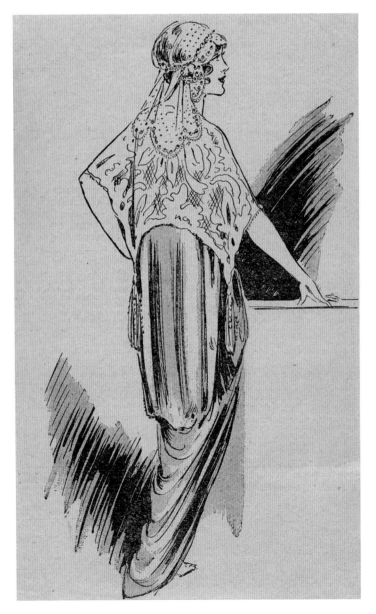

she worked for Redfern or one of the other businesses which were stimulated by the custom of the royal household at Osborne House and visitors to Cowes. Edith married Major Cyril Drummond, from a branch of the Drummonds' banking family, in 1899 and she gave birth to a daughter, Sybelle, in the same year. At the time of the 1911 census, the Drummonds lived in a large house, the Corshams, in Sutton, Surrey, with four domestic servants, including a French lady's maid. In 1960, towards the end of her life, Sybelle made contact with Madeleine Ginsburg in response to an advertisement in *The Times* asking for information about the dressmakers involved with making Heather's wardrobe. Tantalizingly, Sybelle (the Hon. Mrs Sybelle Crossley) referred to a portrait of her mother by Lallie Charles (untraced), and mentioned the fact that her mother was 'rather different from the others ... and did I think introduce some new ideas'.[29]

Mrs Drummond opened her first shop at 29 Church Street, Kensington, in 1903, and Maud Messel (née Sambourne) was a customer.[30] She moved to 89 Park Street in 1907, and a bill headed 'Gowns, hats and blouses' from 1911 made out to Heather at 33 Curzon Street lists four chiffon blouses of a type that Heather seems to have been very fond of. These may have been similar to the blouse with a large Peter Pan collar seen earlier [**39**], gathered in at the waist, with a simple trimming of covered buttons at the centre front, and fringing at the collar and cuffs. From the evidence of a bill dated 7 July 1915 [**128**], Heather was still buying many blouses from Mascotte: these could be refurbished at the shop, which provided new linings and extra collars and cuffs. Mascotte dresses were also available in this distinctive style, with collars and vertical rows of covered buttons in linen and silk [see **30**]; the bills hint at the many other options available in white or blue linen, black or grey charmeuse or taffeta, flowered chiffon and navy striped voile. In 1913, the business had grown, moving a few streets to the east, to 12 and 13 Berkeley Street, off Berkeley Square, and

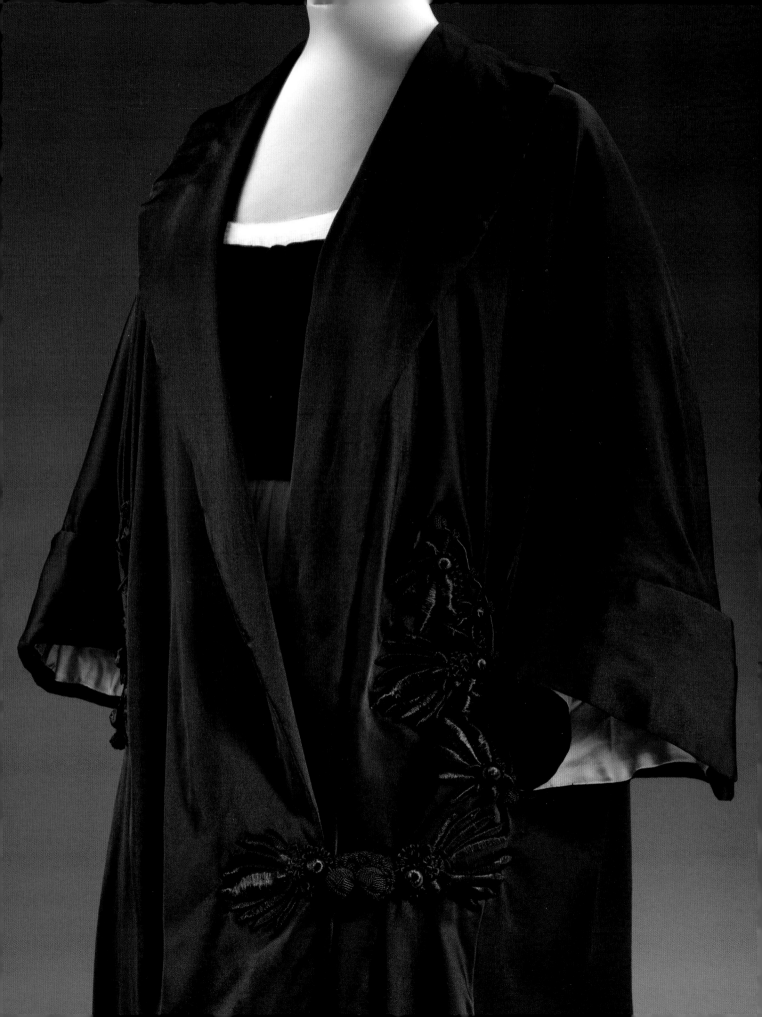

134 Cooper & Machinka, 36 Dover Street, London, *c*.1910
ENGLISH HERITAGE

135 Fashion drawing, Machinka, London, *c*.1922
V&A: HEATHER FIRBANK ARCHIVE

136 Fashion drawing, Machinka, London, *c*.1922
V&A: HEATHER FIRBANK ARCHIVE

137 Bill, Cooper & Machinka, London,
8 January 1907
V&A: HEATHER FIRBANK ARCHIVE

Madame Mascotte's bill announced her headline specialities, now in French, to be 'Robes, Manteaux & Fourrures' [128]. The information on the billhead is framed with a garland of roses and a ribbon, in the contemporary taste for late-eighteenth-century style.

One reason for the low profile of Mascotte could be that there is no evidence the company advertised, although Bessie Ascough does occasionally feature garments from their collections in her fashion reports and these are preserved among Heather's collection of press cuttings. One article features a Mascotte 'Rest Gown' [132], a rather odd-looking garment of pink charmeuse satin with a macramé cape, worn with a boudoir cap. The garment apparently 'sometimes almost merges into a tea gown, so dainty it has become ... it is without exception the most feminine, and becoming garment in our wardrobes', and the article reveals Madame Mascotte 'has a beautiful salon devoted solely to the seduction of negligee tea gowns, blouses and underlinen, and there is no more delightful branch of this great couturière's activities'.[31] The silk evening coat by Mascotte certainly rivals the sophistication and sensuality of Lucile's designs [133].

Apart from a Mascotte gown of about 1906 worn by Maud Messel and now in the collection of Brighton Museum and Art Gallery, no other Mascotte garments have survived in UK museums except for those associated with Heather Firbank.[32] This may be in part because the business lasted for only about 12 years, as at some point during the war Edith Drummond became ill, dying in a nursing home on 27 October 1917. The business closed, and, as had been the fate of Kate Reily's business a decade earlier, the entire stock was bought by Barkers of Kensington, who sold it off at reduced prices from Monday 25 February 1918.[33] A newspaper advertisement published extracts from stock lists, stating 'all garments are up-to-date and with Paris'. Among the most expensive lots listed were two Paris models, an original Doucet coat and skirt in 'Putty Gabardine, trimmed with Navy silk', and a Drecoll coat and skirt in 'Wine Gros-grain'. An elaborate-sounding 'day

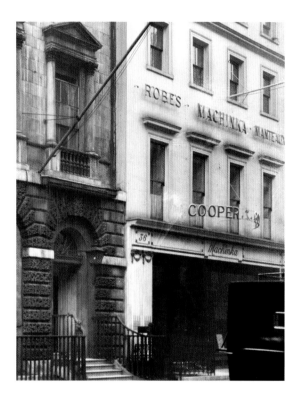

gown in Mole Crêpe Chiffon, trimmed Black silk Net and Lace, waist swathed Gold Tissue', was on sale at 39s 6d (roughly a tenth of the original price, 17½ guineas). Mascotte's trademark rest gowns and wrappers could also be bought greatly reduced, along with chemises, knickers and nightdresses. Home dressmakers could purchase lots from thousands of yards of lace and embroidery – which featured tinsel effects in gold and silver – to rich silks, velvets and dress fabrics including wool coating serges 'the correct weight for Costumes' in saxe, purple, prune, brown and cream.[34] These descriptions in the advertisement illustrated the lavish textiles available even during the war, as dressmakers used up existing stocks.

Mascotte was one of three of Heather's dressmakers (the others were Kate Reily and Charles Lee) to close during or soon after the First World War. The company Machinka, based in Conduit Street from about 1896 (but soon moving to 36 Dover Street, next to Paquin's London base), remained in business

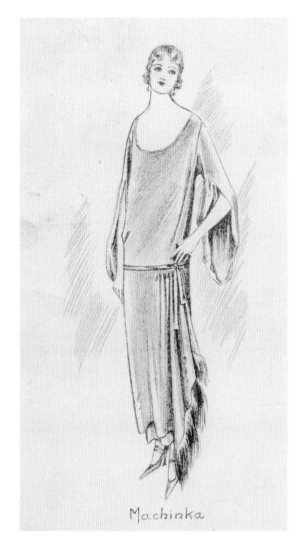

Machinka

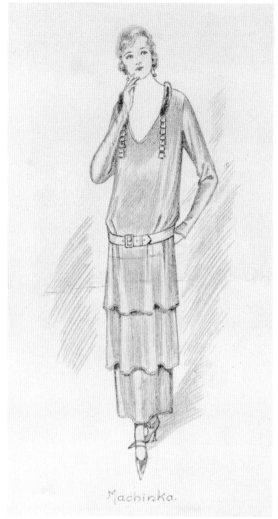

Machinka

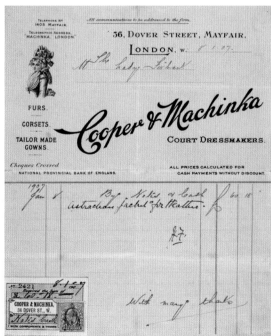

until 1940, although the dressmaker behind the name operated in various partnerships [134]. It was sustained by a reliable group of clients in court circles whose names appear in the descriptions of dresses worn at court published in *The Times*. A bill from Cooper and Machinka dated 8 January 1909 made out to 'The Lady Firbank' charges Heather's mother £60 18s for an 'Astrakhan jacket for Heather', which Lady Firbank paid for with cash, as usual [137]. This is by far the most expensive garment of Heather's, with other furs from the Grafton Fur Company at 164 New Bond Street coming in a close second.

Machinka regularly advertised her return from trips to Paris with the latest fashions.[35] The business operated as the partnership of Cooper and Machinka from about 1904 to 1913. The identity of both, however, remains a mystery, although Machinka is listed among 'many society ladies operating dressmaking businesses under pseudonyms' in 1907, confirming the high status of this dressmaking establishment.[36]

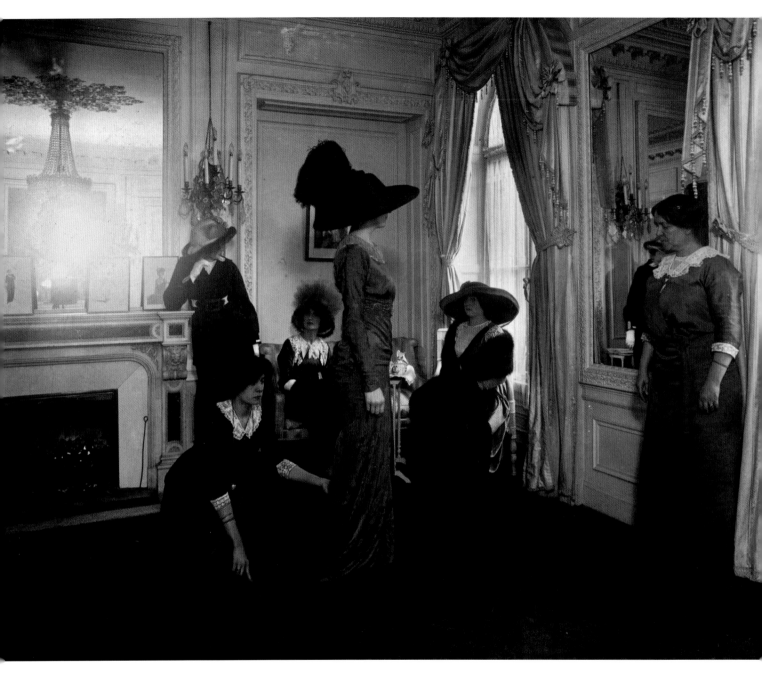

In 1910, the eighteenth-century house, once the home of the Hogarth Club, was remodelled to 'bring the house into accordance with modern business requirements', inserting a wide shop frontage of plate glass framed with marble pilasters that remain in place to this day.[37] The name of Machinka provides an important link in the development of London fashion as one of the firms where the mother of royal dressmaker Hardy Amies (1909–2003) worked as a saleswoman in the early 1900s.[38] Hardy Amies was 'intensely proud' of his connection with the court dressmakers.

A FICTIONAL MILLINER'S SHOP: MADAME DELAINE, PURVEYOR OF MODES, ROBES AND BLOUSES

Business histories of the larger companies are possible to trace through newspaper and magazine reports, but the lack of surviving records has hampered the construction of a history of London's dressmakers, particularly the many smaller businesses and independent concerns. Constance Peel's novel *The Hat Shop*, based on the author's personal experience of running a milliner's shop from about 1908 to 1912, provides a plausible source of information from a businesswoman's point of view. Despite its occasionally moralistic tone and some stereotypical characters, the novel illuminates the circumstances in which fashionable clothing in London was produced. The heroine, recently widowed Elizabeth Earl, is a tall, slight woman of thirty-four 'dressed in extreme simplicity in well-cut blue serge'. She sets up shop with 'spotless white paint and gilt lettering' in a Knightsbridge street as Madame Delaine, 'Purveyor of Modes, Robes, et Blouses'. Just as Henry Mayhew described in his account of dressmaking businesses in the 1840s in *London Labour and the London Poor*, Madame Delaine's shop was converted from a four-storey family home.[39] A large shop window had replaced the original window, with the hall, front and back rooms connected with arches. The showrooms were plainly furnished, in contrast to the carefully constructed interiors created earlier by Lady Duff-Gordon at Lucile:

White papered walls almost hidden by white framed looking-glasses, white chairs, a green carpeted floor, and a couple of small white dressing tables with swing mirror, hand mirror, huge lace and flower trimmed pincushion, together with some thirty white enamelled millinery stands on which were arranged hats of every description, completed the furnishing of the millinery showroom.[40]

There was a fitting room on the half-landing, and a second showroom and a second fitting room with electric light for trying on evening wear on the next floor. On the top floor were workrooms for the head milliner and her assistants, and separate skirt and bodice workrooms run by the cutter and fitter. These had whitewashed walls, which were hung with large documents provided by the Home Office listing recently issued rules to be observed in workrooms, and were furnished with long deal tables and wooden chairs, and speaking tubes connecting workroom with showrooms and office.

These rooms were warmed by gas stoves on which irons were heating, and a faint smell caused by hot metal passing over damp material and by the paste and wet sparterie [a fine pliable mesh woven out of willow fibres that is better quality than buckram and suitable for large brims] used by the milliners pervaded the upper part of the house, while a slight vibration and low hum of sound proclaimed the presence of the treadle sewing machine.

The basement housed the girls' meal room, where 'frugal tea provided by the house was dispensed, and those girls who could not afford to lunch at restaurants, however humble, cooked and ate their midday meal, and on wet days read their novelettes in the dinner hour'.[41]

A rare glimpse of milliners in their working environment is shown in a series of photographs taken by Bassano Ltd of Old Bond Street in 1910 for the hat makers Maison Lewis, who retailed from large showrooms just south of Oxford Circus, and also operated Louise & Co. on Regent Street [**139, 140**]. This company is not represented among Heather's surviving collection of hats, although a single bill suggests that she did make at least one purchase at this successful British company, which also had branches in Paris and Monte Carlo. Women who worked as milliners looked down on dressmakers[42] and they could often earn a very good living, as is shown by a report on a 1913 court case which describes the attributes required of milliners who progressed to become showroom assistants:

[they] must have natural tastes and adaptability ... intimate knowledge of changing fashions; fine taste for colour combination; ability to model and design; an attractive and convincing method with customers ... Personality means a good deal ... we often have customers who insist on seeing one special assistant or department manageress ... In the case of hats two persons are rarely similar. For one thing, the trimming is expected to suit the complexion; while the size of the hats [is] largely dictated by the contour of the face.[43]

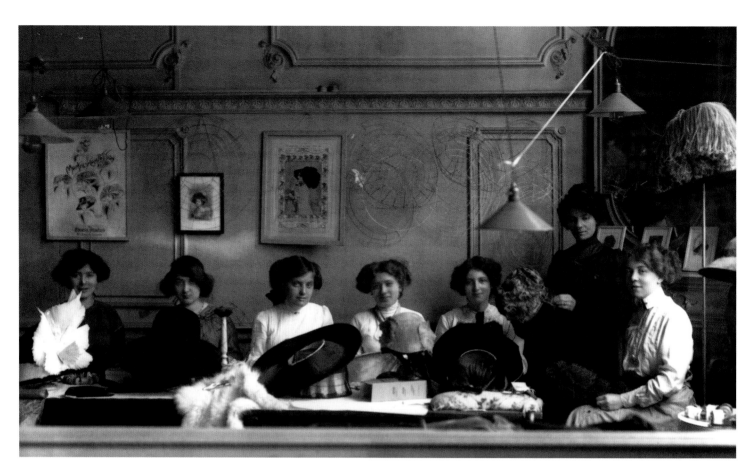

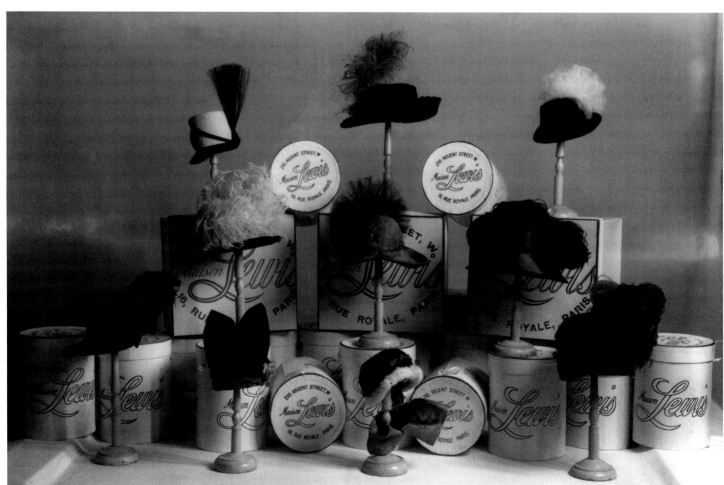

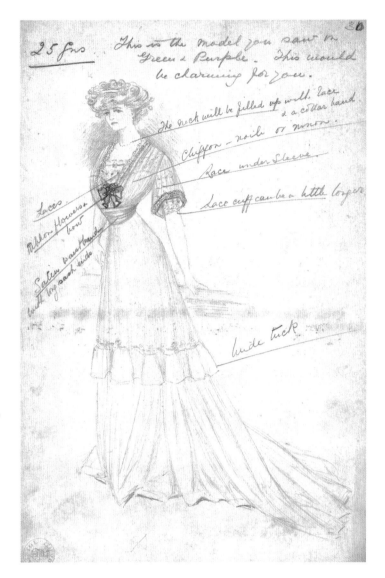

This illustrates the kind of personal skills required of the thousands of milliners and dressmakers working in London's thriving retail industry in the pre-war period. There are no details of the inter-actions between wealthy customers such as Heather Firbank and showroom staff, but bills and other documents in her archive and extracts from mem-oirs written by her contemporaries illustrate the process of buying a dress, from choosing to fitting and delivery.

'THIS WOULD BE CHARMING FOR YOU': SHOPPING AT A COURT DRESSMAKER

Among Heather's papers are two pencil sketches showing dresses of the early 1920s by Machinka of Dover Street [**135, 136**], and these are likely to have been some of many that were sent to her to choose from or perhaps taken home after a fashion show for further consideration. These could be annotated with explanations or suggestions of material, and with adaptations to suit clients' particular requirements. Copies of sketches in the Lucile archive have the following written on the reverse: 'Unless returned within 2 days, the sum of 7/6 will be charged for this sketch.'[44] This warning may have become necessary because of the tendency of unscrupulous clients to take a sketch to a cheaper dressmaker to have it copied.

The famous fashion shows held at Lucile were a brilliant way of selling designs to already willing customers. Naturally Heather attended these shows and those of other London court dressmakers. A 'Programme of models' from Lucile, dated Spring 1923 [**142**], survives in her papers, listing 77 designs, some given evocative names, such as '*Mon Réve*' (My Dream), a 'fawn rep one-piece dress'; 'Wind o' the Water', a black and silver tea gown, and 'Garden of Roses', a 'silver brocaded evening gown', which Heather marked with a tick. Heather had ticked 7 out of the 77 models shown at this fashion show: a day gown of black moracain (a type of silk), an afternoon gown, a tea gown, three evening gowns and a black

velvet cloak. This fashion show programme clearly shows Heather's active interest in fashion in 1923, at the age of 35, though there is no evidence that she ever ordered any of these dresses.

After a fashion show or at a later appointment, a vendeuse (senior saleswoman) or perhaps the designer herself would assist in agreeing any adapta-tions to the design and making a final decision. A pencil sketch in the Lucile archive demonstrates the process [**141**]. Headed 'This is the model you saw in green and purple. This one would be charming for you', the design is annotated with comments such as 'Satin waistband with long sash ends' and 'The neck will be filled up with lace and a collar band'. These notes would have helped the customer visualize the final dress and reassured her that it would not com-promise her need for modesty. Once she had decided, she would have returned a few days later for a fitting,

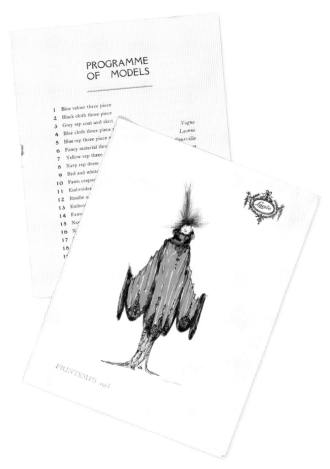

which could be a tedious process. Cynthia Asquith described the experience as

endless wearisome hours of trying-on. Shifting my weight from one foot to another, I stood twitching with boredom while portentously solemn women, with their mouths full of pins, and tape-measures slung around their necks, knelt on my feet, conferring with one another and from time to time appealing to the not wholly attentive lady of the house.[45]

Once fitted a dress would be made up by the different specialist seamstresses, with separate bodice and skirt hands, and embroidery completed by another highly skilled specialist. The dress would be delivered a short time later to the client's home in a dress box. For particularly demanding and inconsiderate clients, dresses, even complicated and elaborate court dresses, could be delivered in a matter of hours. A letter in the V&A files about the *Lady of Fashion* exhibition from a dressmaker who worked at Mascotte states that dresses were packed in plain brown cardboard boxes, while court dresses would be packed in a large black leather box with the dressmaker's name on it.[46] Subsequently, the dressmaker's book-keeper would send a bill – often once several garments had been ordered and delivered, from the evidence of Heather's papers. Many wealthy and well-known customers were notoriously bad at paying their bills, but Heather (or usually her brother Ronald) paid her bills sometimes as soon as three days after they were issued, and she received a 10 per cent discount for paying in cash. Heather would have been a highly valued customer and her dressmakers entered into long-standing relationships with her. Bills such as one sent from Mascotte in 1915 show that the company offered a complete service, including refurbishment, cleaning and repairs to garments [128]. This made the investment in couture clothes more worthwhile for the customer, and it was probably cost-effective for the dressmaker to offer this service as labour costs were low.

All women, of all ages, who moved in these upper-class circles spent many hours with dressmakers and other specialist suppliers. Some, like Heather, would have found it an absorbing and creative process. Cynthia Asquith, however, remembered that at the age of 17, 'clothes represented the extremes of boredom and delight. I hated "trying-on" in the dreary embryonic pin and holland-foundation stage, but revelled in the excitement of an all-but finished new dress and the thrill of buying something ready-to-wear'.[47] She was among a new generation of debutantes who were prepared to buy clothing already made up, albeit from the grandest of London department stores and for everyday rather than evening functions.

DEPARTMENT STORES

The status of large department stores had improved through the second part of the nineteenth century and many, such as Debenham & Freebody, expanded from a traditional drapery business with roots in the eighteenth century, setting up their own workrooms to compete with the court dressmakers and attract the 'carriage class' – those, like Heather's family, who owned or could afford to hire their own means of

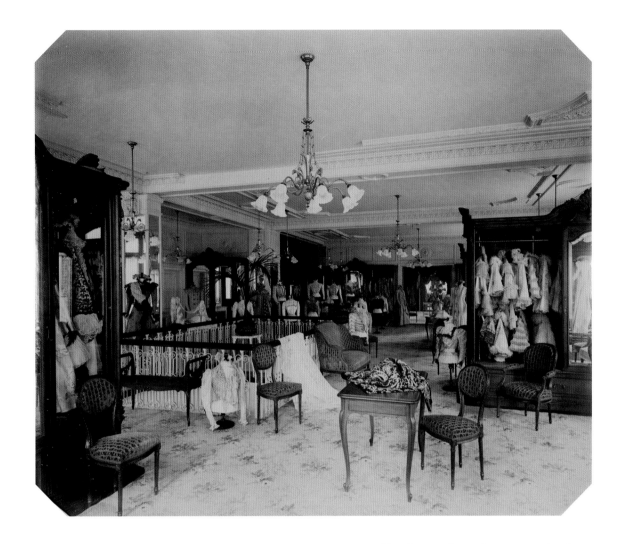

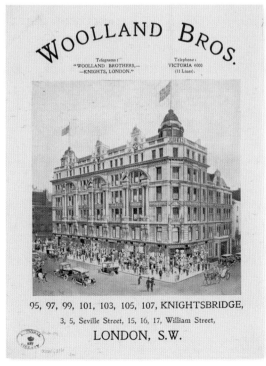

transport. The first ready-made garments in about 1850 were loose mantles, cloaks and shawls, which avoided the need for time-consuming personal fittings, but through mail order and initiatives such as selling partially made bodices and skirts, Oxford Street department stores such as Peter Robinson and Marshall & Snelgrove became the first manufacturers of ready-made fashion. Heather's bills show that she bought much of her underwear and blouses ready-made in this way, particularly from the exclusive department store Woolland Brothers in Knightsbridge. She regularly received deliveries of other garments, such as petticoats and hats, from Woollands on approval, sent to her at the Coopers in Kent to choose from by shop assistants who must have known her taste well [145].[48]

Demolished in 1969, Woollands once stood on the site of the current Sheraton Park Tower hotel, next door to the department store Harvey Nichols [144]. At the end of the nineteenth century Woollands was the epitome of respectable high-class Victorian

1909

May June						
			To a/c rendered		82	15	8
June 23	1	White Petticoat		2	3	9
	1	Cotton			9	6
	1	" "			16	9
	1	Green Knickers			12	9
26	6	Vests	1/6	3	3	0
29	1	White Night Gown		2	17	9
	1	White Corsets		2	2	0
	1	" "		4	4	0
30	5	Chemises	13/9	3	3	9
	2	"	11/9	1	3	6
	3	"	9/10	1	9	9
	2	"	10/9	1	1	6
	2	"	11/6	1	3	0
	2	"	9/11		19	10
	1	"			14	9
	1	"			14	6
	2	"	19/6	1	19	0
	1	Knickers			8	9
	2	"	19/6	1	1	0
	2	"	19/6	1	1	0
	2	White Silk Petticoats	33/9	3	7	6
	1	Nainsook "		1	17	9
	1	"		2	9	6
	1	"		1	1	9
		Carried forward		122	14	0

145 Bill, Woolland Brothers, London, July 1909
V&A: HEATHER FIRBANK ARCHIVE

146 A group of single gloves, France, *c.*1910 (from left to right): day glove, antelope leather, evening glove, kid leather, retailed by Augustus Bide, London, day glove, antelope leather, day glove, leather, retailed by Frederick Penberthy, London
V&A: T.84–1960, T.79–1960, T.75–1960, T.81–1960

retailing, supplying the residents of Belgravia and Mayfair and visitors from further afield with 'dressmaking in all its branches', and 'ladies tailoring and family mourning' through 22 different departments, including furnishing fabrics and haberdashery. The Woolland brothers, Samuel and William from Bridford in Devon, started in 1869 by taking over a single draper's shop at Lowndes Terrace. Two decades later the family business had subsumed six adjoining shops, eventually completing an entire rebuilding project resulting in a steel-framed construction faced in Portland stone, with a continuous run of plateglass windows. An interior view of the first-floor showrooms from the 1890s shows open cupboards displaying capes and jackets, with small chairs and tables arranged to invite customers to rest and consider potential purchases [143]. The showrooms were on the ground and first floors, with workrooms on the next two floors and kitchen, dining rooms and assistants' sitting rooms on the upper floors. Sleeping accommodation for staff was located in nearby lodging houses.[49] At the turn of the nineteenth century the company enjoyed the custom of aristocrats such as the Duchess of Portland and Edward VII's mistress Alice Keppel, who would bring her daughters down from Edinburgh four times a year to shop at Woollands (see p.16). Heather may have visited the Juvenile Department at the same time; she was certainly loyal to the store, continuing to buy hats from there while living in Hove in her fifties, as a bill from June 1940 shows.[50]

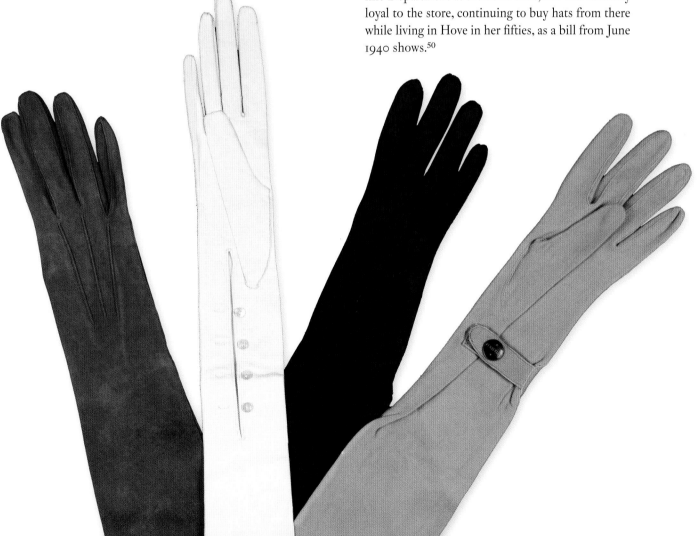

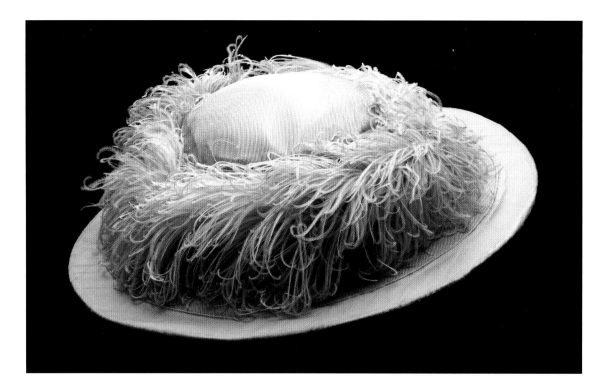

In addition to hats and underwear, Heather also favoured their tailoring, as a labelled tailor-made costume of about 1910 attests [147, 148]. Made out of the urban standby navy-blue serge, but with a striking collar and triangular skirt panel of striped blanket-type cloth, this costume may have been worn for travelling or for walking while away from London rather than for 'street' wear in Mayfair or Belgravia.

TRADITIONAL SPECIALITY SHOPS
While some family businesses, such as Woolland Brothers and Debenham & Freebody, flourished and expanded their clientele with the growing middle classes, other more specialist suppliers stayed close to their traditional roots. Heather relied on these smaller businesses for specialized accessories, including hats, gloves and shoes: for example, she bought many of her large quantity of soft felt hats and straw boaters for wearing in the country and for sports from the hatters Woodrow & Sons of 46 Piccadilly.[51] Equally essential were gloves, which were needed to complete every outfit, from fine cream kid gloves covering the arms for evening wear to heavier 'gauntlets' or gloves with deep cuffs to wear for walking, shopping, travel or sport [146]. A bill from Augustus Bide of New Bond Street reveals the great variety of colours and hides available – and the quantities Heather required in order to maintain her appearance. The bill lists a total of 44 pairs of gloves which Heather bought on

147 Hat, covered with ribbed silk and trimmed with ostrich feathers, Woolland Brothers, 1908–10
V&A: CIRC.650-1964

three occasions from 20 July to 29 September 1909, including five pairs of white kid gloves, one of which cost £1 2s 6d, the most expensive gloves on the bill. Other types of animal skins used included coloured antelope, white doe and 'beaver coloured' reindeer. Augustus Bide's company began trading at North Audley Street in 1847 and continued to operate in the Mayfair area until the Second World War. Stamped labels inside some of Heather's gloves show that they were made in France, which was known for producing high-quality accessories. She bought one pair from Debenham & Freebody.

The Heather Firbank Collection includes 14 pairs of shoes, ranging from robust tan leather boots for country walking to buttoned boots of patent leather and suede for city use [149-55]. There are also Louis-heeled 'Langtry' shoes decorated with a self-coloured buckle; laced 'Oxfords' in suede and leather; and glamorous court shoes for evening wear in purple leather, white and gold, and a single stunning pair of gold court shoes. From the evidence of the stamped labels in the lining of the shoes and three surviving bills, Heather bought her shoes from three shops: Hook, Knowles & Co., Alan McAfee and the enterprising court dressmaker Charles Lee of Wigmore Street (1890–1913) and Sloane Street

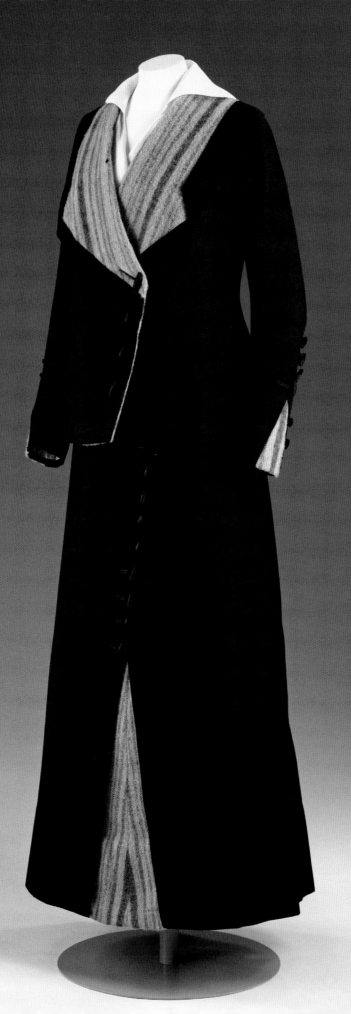

148 Tailored walking costume
(jacket and skirt), wool serge
with blanket wool, Woolland
Brothers, London, *c.*1910

V&A: T.37&A-1960

(1906–10), who, unusually, included shoes in the specialities listed on his bill. Charles Lee – who built up a wide range of products from his initial specialism as a 'court hosier and glover', as listed in the Post Office directories – actively promoted his business in the press and, unlike Heather's other dressmakers, who perhaps saw themselves as above this need to reach new customers, took part in an exhibition of Paris and London fashion in Earls Court in January 1908.[52] One notice in the press boasted: 'Mr. Lee has his workrooms in such condition and so admirably controlled that he is in a position to undertake any orders for evening gowns and tailor-mades at the shortest possible notice.'[53] Mr Lee also brought attention to the fact that he displayed evening wear in artificial light,[54] and he was among a few other dressmakers who marketed 'Suffragette' fashions in the colours of white, green and purple.[55]

From Lee's extensive shop at 26–29 Sloane Street, Heather bought two pairs of her very glamorous gold court shoes for the high price of £1 13s 6d, along with two pairs of silver court shoes and pairs of silk hose in gold, silver and white in May 1909 [51]. Most of her shoes, however, were supplied by two Mayfair family businesses, Hook, Knowles & Co. (established in 1842 in New Bond Street), which supplied the royal family [149, 150, 152, 154], and Alan McAfee, which opened in 1898 at 68 Duke Street and remained in business at various addresses until 1989. A bill of 1909 from Alan McAfee lists seven pairs of Langtry shoes in green, brown, grey and violet 'seal' at £2 10s a pair [151, 153, 155]. Alan McAfee also traded as Alan's Shoes, and opened a new shop at 237 Regent Street in the summer of 1915, selling shoes made in the company's off-site factory. With rising hemlines, 'footgear has been playing a large and ever increasing part in the ensemble of the fashionably dressed woman', as a newspaper report announced. Staff were maintained on the premises to make to order when required, and it is possible that many of Heather's shoes were custom-made by the company's London-based shoemakers.[56]

THE SHOP GIRL

In 1909, according to the 47 surviving bills for that year, Heather spent over £1,063, more than twice the annual allowance of £525 that she would eventually receive. Letters from a decade later, when the family's financial situation had deteriorated further, show that Heather's expenses caused a great deal of concern to her mother and brother, and she continued to overspend on a large scale. However, Heather was not the only young woman who needed additional financial help from her family. Cynthia Asquith was given a chequebook and £100 a year to spend on her wardrobe. She recalled: 'So many different kinds of clothes were considered necessary and my hunting outfit made a large extra.' She was 17 and felt 'illimitably rich' but soon found herself 'chronically overdrawn'.[57]

Despite the vast size of Heather's surviving wardrobe, even taking into account the additional lots sold at Christie's in 1974, there are clearly many garments missing, as none of the descriptions in the bills match up definitively with surviving dresses or accessories. This adds up to an impossibly large wardrobe for most of us today, but Heather's shopping habits have to be seen in the context of society's expectations at the time. As a smart, well-brought-up woman 'out' in society she would have changed her clothing several times throughout the day, with the help of her personal maid, Hallett.

The cost of just one of Heather's many silk evening dresses [112] listed at £25 4s was almost as much as the £26 a year or 10 shillings a week that many 'hands' in dress and millinery workshops could expect to earn before 1914.[58] Admittedly, pay and conditions in the high-class dressmaking establishments, such as those supplying Heather, were comparatively good, and according to a widely reported employment tribunal of 1913, a skilled West End dressmaker would be in demand and could earn up to £300 a year.[59] These figures illustrate the scale of Heather's expenditure on her wardrobe in relation to the earnings of the working classes, many of whom depended on this lavish spending. A variety of sources, such

149 Court shoe, kid leather, Hook, Knowles & Co., London, *c.*1910
V&A: T.143–1960

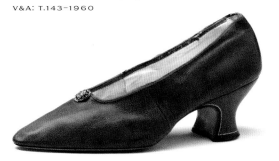

150 Walking boot, leather, Hook, Knowles & Co., London, *c.*1908
V&A: T.148–1960

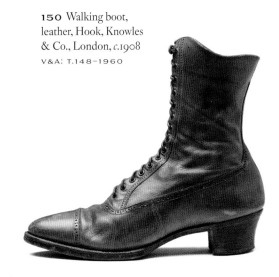

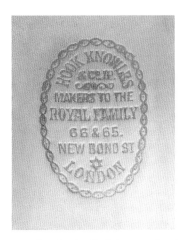

152 Interior detail of plate 154 showing stamped maker's name

151 Boots, kid leather and suede, Alan McAfee, *c.*1914
V&A: CIRC.660&A–1964

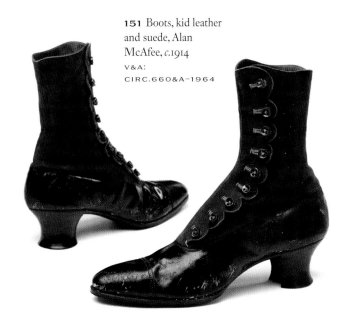

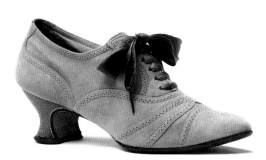

153 Oxford shoe, suede, Alan McAfee, London, *c.*1914
V&A: T.137–1960

154 Evening court shoes, kid leather, Hook, Knowles & Co., London, *c.*1910
V&A: T.150&A–1960

155 'Langtry' shoe, purple suede leather, Alan McAfee, London, *c.*1910–14
V&A: T.149–1960

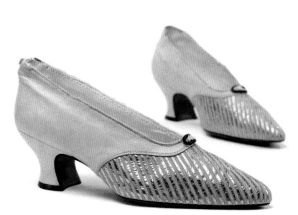

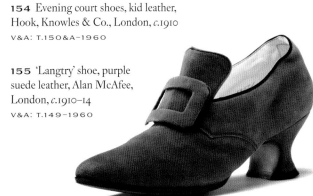

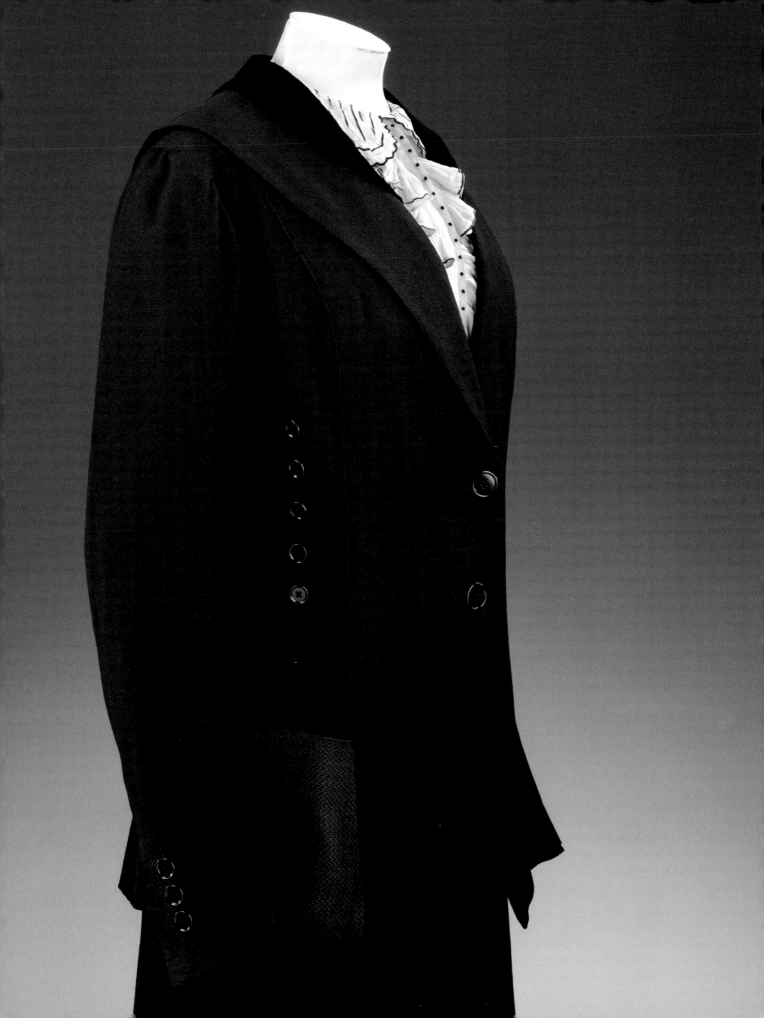

as Constance Peel's novel *The Hat Shop* and the
detailed evidence of the Charles Booth surveys of
the 1890s, suggest that in some ways dressmaking
establishments of the early twentieth century had
not changed drastically from those described by
Henry Mayhew 60 years earlier, although consum-
ers were well aware of the poor living conditions of
many working in the garment trades. Philanthropists,
socialists and feminist groups mounted separate efforts to study pay and conditions, develop trade
unions in all branches of the industry, and suggest so-
lutions to the exploitation of overworked, underpaid
needlewomen.[60] These campaigns eventually forced
Parliament to set up the Select Committee on the
Sweating System (1888–90). The most public dem-
onstration of concern was focused on the 1906 *Daily
News* 'Sweated Industries Exhibition' at the Queen's
Hall, Bayswater, part of the trend for educational and
spectacular exhibitions. However, it was not until the
Trade Board acts of 1909 and 1918 that progress was
made in restricting long working days and regulat-
ing wages, by which time the war and the continuing
development of factories had greatly simplified clothing and its production.

The bills and documents in the Heather Firbank
archive, while offering an insight into the identity of
Heather's Mayfair dressmakers and the pricing of
fashionable dress in the period, reveal little about
the lives of the individuals concerned in its manufac-
ture. A single undated, handwritten letter, on paper
with a printed heading of 'Lucie, Corsetière' of 40,
Sternhold Avenue, Streatham Hill, SW2, is an exception: from 'Lucie' herself, it explains that she has
just left Lucile of Hanover Square, where she was
head corsetière for several years, 'well-remembering
[Heather's] name'. Having over 17 years of practical
experience at this specialist skill, Lucie offers to make
corsets in 'pretty and durable material from 2 guineas per pair', and suggests that she would call upon
Heather in town to fit, or could copy one of her existing corsets. Unfortunately, there is no strong evidence
from the census and local street directories to help

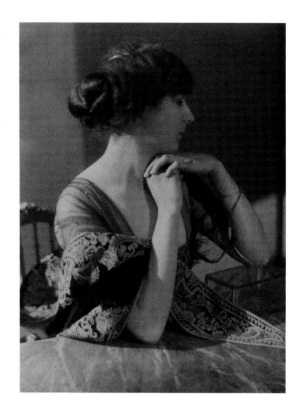

identify Lucie's real name, as she was using the association with her previous employer to help launch
herself as a private corsetière in her local community.

One of Heather's two surviving corsets [**26**] is
marked with a faint name and address, very likely
that of 'Mesdames Devalois & Rocher, Corsetières
de Paris', of 59 Beauchamp Place, whose business
card is kept with Heather's papers. Directories show
the shop in operation from 1915 to 1930, although it
likely opened earlier, moving to 34 Beauchamp Place,
Brompton Road, in the early 1920s. The existence of
such 'Corsetières de Paris' in London confirms the
strong association of the quality of fit and correct aesthetic with corsets made in Paris or by those who had
apparently trained there. While genuine individuals
corresponding to the names 'Devalois & Rocher'
cannot be found in the census or Post Office directories, the listing for the company in 1918 does give
the names 'Mme M. Meunier & Mlle S. Gathier'.

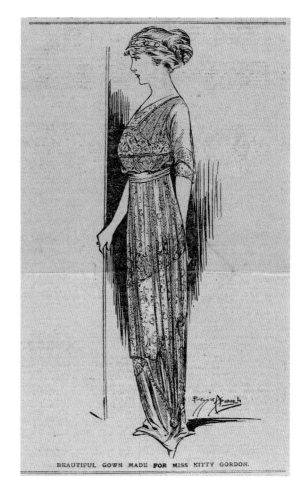

BEAUTIFUL GOWN MADE FOR MISS KITTY GORDON.

A Suzanne Gathier, daughter of Louis Gathier, a clerk in a general merchant's office, of Loughborough Road, Brixton, is listed in the 1911 census as a corset maker's apprentice, and her sister Marguerite seems to have joined the business, eventually becoming the sole proprietor of Devalois & Rocher. This example suggests that French residents in London took advantage of their connections with Paris, the ultimate source of fashion, alongside British women who encouraged perceptions of themselves as having similar French credentials. The frequency of French and other nationals occupied in dressmaking or associated trades listed in boarding houses in the census of 1911 furthermore suggests that London, perhaps unsurprisingly, was seen as fertile ground for opportunities in fashion.

The dramatic disparity between the lives of the young women who made fine clothes in the West End and those of the more fortunate women who wore them was attacked and explored to dramatic and popular effect in a whole genre of musical comedies – effectively 'rags to riches' stories – which were produced at playhouses such as the Gaiety Theatre, including *The Shop Girl* (1895) and *Warp and Woof* (1904). The London stage at the same time fuelled demand for the latest fashions by providing London dressmakers with a vital platform to advertise their work. Public awareness of the interdependency of theatre and fashion at this time is clearly expressed in an article from Heather's fashion cuttings showing a 'Quartet of Charming Gowns' made for actress Miss Kitty Gordon by Mascotte, one of Heather's favourite dressmakers [158].

To many women the stage represents a walk down Bond-street and a visit to the Rue de la Paix rolled into one. Very often the loveliest dresses make their appearance behind the footlights, and the woman who pays a visit to the theatre often does so with a double intention of profiting by the latest fashion news, as well as amusing herself vastly by the play.[61]

Recent studies of the overlapping worlds of fashion and popular theatre have explored the role of London's musicals and drawing-room dramas in promoting dressmaking houses and new trends in fashion and interiors, while fuelling the aspirations of the middle classes.[62] The stars of London's stages, such as Lily Elsie and Gaby Deslys, were certainly a fruitful source of inspiration for those growing up in the pre-war era, such as Norman Hartnell, who would become London's best-known couturier of the twentieth century.[63]

Another image from Heather's collection of magazine cuttings, from the *Sketch* supplement of 1913, shows the strikingly modern appearance and attitude of a London shop girl [159]. All *Sketch* readers would have understood the reference to the 'Shop Girl' as the title of the popular play. This reproduction of a portrait by Harold Speed shows a Lucile employee, in a slim, plain, almost shapeless coat and skirt, carrying a distinctive green and white dress box [160]. While Heather's own tailor-made costumes of this time might have indicated her high status and wealth through the quality of cloth and subtle details of trim, the image of the

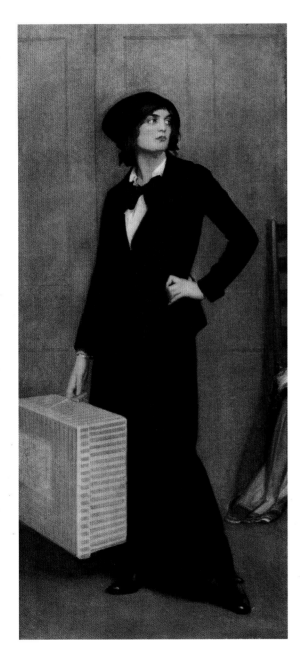

shop girl suggests a force of change seen on the streets of London, with the traditional authorities of fashionable dress yielding to the pressures of the modern world.

Heather Firbank's wardrobe and the papers that survive with the clothes open up a view of the dressmakers of Mayfair, where luxury clothes were designed, fitted and made, sustaining a network of creativity and expertise which, a century later, still supports the British and international designers retailing from their shops in the streets between Bond Street and Dover Street and the surrounding area. In the words of Constance Peel, Edwardian English women were 'apt to overdress and to be untidy ... and often spoilt the effect of a good dress and hat by an ill-chosen handbag or the wrong stockings or gloves', while 'French women, then as now, dressed quietly for the street. Their neatness was exquisite and every detail of the toilette was carefully thought out.'[64] The exquisitely dressed Heather Firbank exhibited these exact qualities, and showed definitively that London dressmakers could compete with the best that Paris had to offer.

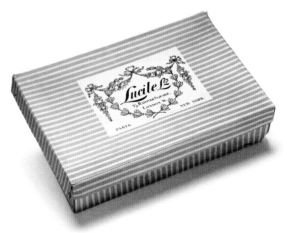

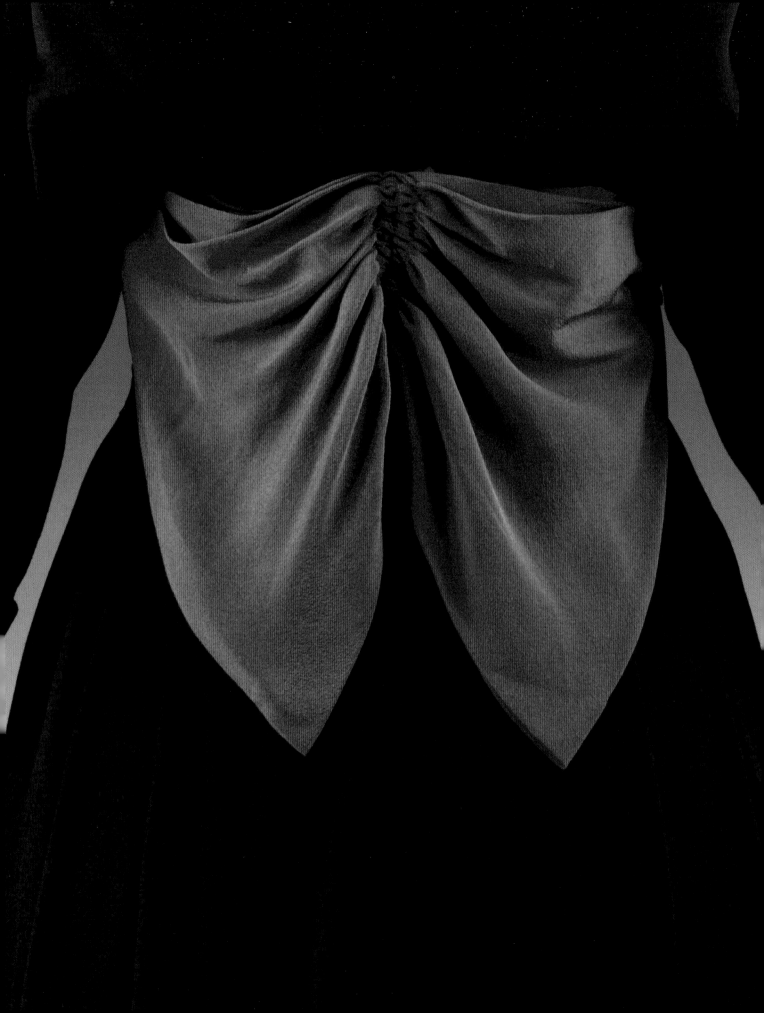

CONCLUSION

This capsule of one woman's wardrobe provides a snapshot of changing fashions and, importantly, Heather Firbank's changing personal style in the formative years of her life. By reuniting the clothes with the story of their wearer we can see how the collection traces her emergence into London society, the blossoming of her interest in fashion and experimentation with more risqué styles, and her retreat to safer territory and a wardrobe that reflected the isolation of her later life. What survives reveals the preoccupations of a woman moving in society circles in the decade before the First World War, her need to conform to specific codes of dressing for different times of day and various social events, and the importance of maintaining a fashionable appearance within etiquette-appropriate boundaries.

Throughout the changes in fashion and in her lifestyle there is a consistency to Heather's choices that makes her clothes easy to distinguish among the vast collections at the V&A. Heather's clothes are never the most showy or the most obviously fashionable. Instead, she favoured an understated elegance: an exquisitely tailored Lucile jacket with a bright silk lining, a selection of evening dresses and daywear in muted tones of purple and grey, and near-identical blouses bought in multiples of the same design in different colours. She always patronized London couturiers and avoided more avant-garde, artistic dressmakers. A strong identity emerges from these clothing choices and from the surviving letters: Heather was a bold image maker who, born into wealth, was absorbed by and entirely unable to resist the temptations of luxury fashion.

As a consequence of this absorption, Heather has left us today with a truly remarkable and precious dress collection. Her wardrobe and associated bills and ephemera offer a unique opportunity to study the creative talents of London fashion, shoe and hat designers of this period, and to admire and learn about the remarkable manufacturing skills of the anonymous army of seamstresses, tailors, shoemakers and milliners who made her beautiful clothes. This case study has pulled Heather as a living, breathing personality out from the shadow of her more famous brother, Ronald, and also from the shadow of her own famous dress collection at the V&A. As Heather instinctively understood, clothes are an expression of an individual's personality and personal choices. In the words of one of her favourite dressmakers, Lucile, 'I always saw the woman, not the frock as detached from her ... because women are above all other things personal in every thought and action.'[1]

In its personal, biographical elements, this case study reflects a wider trend in historical research, focusing on individuals and their stories to reveal new perspectives on the past. In *Historiography in the Twentieth Century* (2005), Professor George G. Iggers has written: 'Not history but histories, or better stories, are what matter now.'[2] Heather's story matters. This more personal approach is also evident in the proliferation of fashion exhibitions over the last decade dedicated to showing one woman's wardrobe. Whether these showcase the fashion choices of a well-known individual such as Queen Maud or Jackie Kennedy or of somebody less well known such as Jill Ritblat and Mrs Tinne, the intention is that through these more personal displays histories and memories will meet and that a more emotive experience will ultimately be achieved, leading to a deeper understanding of the past.[3]

161 Afternoon dress (back detail of plate 36)

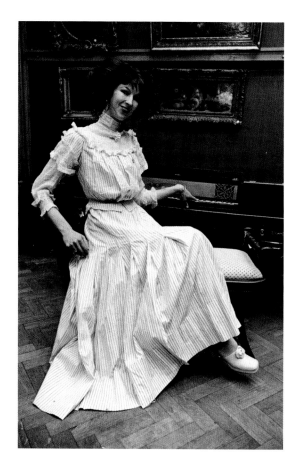

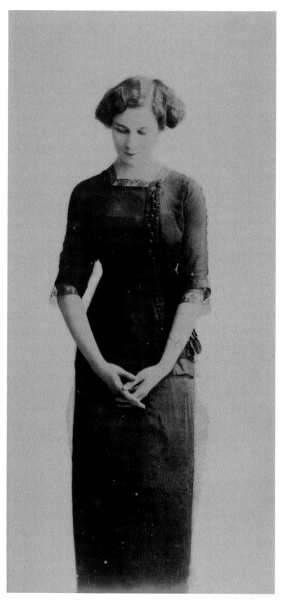

162 Johanna Firbank wearing a Heather Firbank dress, 1974
V&A: HEATHER FIRBANK ARCHIVE

163 Heather Firbank, photographed by Rita Martin,
London, *c.*1912
V&A: HEATHER FIRBANK ARCHIVE

'A LIFE BEYOND HER OWN LIFE'

There is an addendum to this story in that Heather's family have continued to enjoy the use of items of Heather's wardrobe that did not find their way into museum collections. Heather's nephew, Lieutenant-Colonel Thomas Firbank, wore one of Ronald's broad-striped summer blazers, while his wife dressed in one of Heather's gowns at a family fancy-dress party in the 1960s. His daughter, Johanna Firbank (Heather's great-niece), remembers that she never had to worry about evening clothes because Heather's not only fitted her well but, in their 'classic' style, were perfect for late 1960s fashions [162]. In 1971, she was married wearing an adapted white silk Heather Firbank dress and wore Heather's Burberry mackintosh on walks in the Welsh countryside.[4]

Whether cherished and worn by the family or displayed and researched as invaluable examples of historical fashionable dress in museums around the UK, these garments have continued to be valued and held in the same high regard that their original owner bestowed on them. It is fitting that Johanna Firbank, understanding all of this so well, should provide the last word to this book. She commented that Heather valued her clothes as 'works of art' and that they 'now have a life beyond her own life' – as inspirational garments, exhibited, studied and admired in the Museum.[5]

APPENDIX:
HEATHER FIRBANK GARMENTS
IN UK COLLECTIONS

1905–8

*c.***1905** Summer day dress (plate 17). Blue and white striped cotton trimmed with broderie anglaise, machine lace and pearl buttons.
Maker unknown, British
V&A: T.21A-C-1960

*c.***1905** Nightdress. White linen with green ribbon and embroidery.
Maker unknown, British
V&A: T.68-1960

*c.***1905** Drawers (plate 20). Pale pink silk with embroidered 'Heather' motif and machine lace inserts.
Maker unknown, British
V&A: T.71-1960

*c.***1905** Petticoat. Cream flannel with machine embroidery.
Maker unknown, British
GALLERY OF COSTUME, MANCHESTER: 1963.309

*c.***1905** Petticoat. White cotton trimmed with embroidery and green ribbon.
Maker unknown, British
GALLERY OF COSTUME, MANCHESTER: 1963.310

1905–8 Golfing ensemble (plate 69). Tailored jacket, skirt and cap, brown and black striped 'homespun' tweed and tan leather.
Frederick Bosworth, London
V&A: T.20A-D-1960

*c.***1906** Summer day dress. Mauve and white striped cotton voile.
Maker unknown, British
MUSEUM OF LONDON: 74.37/6

*c.***1906** Petticoat. White cotton trimmed with pink silk ribbon and machine embroidery.
Maker unknown, British
V&A: T.67-1960

*c.***1906** Combinations. Cream wool.
Marshall and Snelgrove, London
V&A: T.134-1960

1906–8 Hat. Straw boater with cream silk band.
Lucile, London
V&A: T.117-1960

1907–8 Motoring coat. Cream wool twill with mauve cloth trim.
Woolland Brothers, London
MUSEUM OF LONDON: 74.37/7

*c.***1908** Tailored jacket and skirt (plate 31). Lilac-grey wool trimmed with silk braid, lined with silk satin.
Frederick Bosworth, London
V&A: T.26&A-1960

*c.***1908** Summer day dress (plate 28). Pink linen trimmed with machine lace and machine embroidery.
Maker unknown, British
V&A: T.22&A-1960

*c.***1908** Tailored jacket and skirt (plate 32). Navy-blue wool serge trimmed with black braid.
Redfern, London
V&A: CIRC.646&A-1964

*c.***1908** Purple silk handkerchiefs with embroidered 'Heather' motif.
Probably Redfern, London
V&A: T.42B&C-1960

*c.***1908** Blouse (plate 38). White cotton lawn with machine lace and hand-worked embroidery.
Maker unknown, British
V&A: T.59-1960

*c.***1908** Hat (plate 3). Cream straw with silk flowers.
Woolland Brothers, London
V&A: T.103-1960

*c.***1908** Blouse. Black and white striped cotton lawn.
Irish Linen Stores, London
V&A: CIRC.648-1964

*c.***1908** Blouse. Red and white striped cotton lawn.
Irish Linen Stores, London
MUSEUM OF LONDON: 74.37/9

*c.***1908** Blouse. Green and white striped cotton lawn.
Irish Linen Stores, London
GALLERY OF COSTUME, MANCHESTER: 1963.304

1908–10

1908–10 Corset. Cream silk with silk satin ribbon, elasticated suspenders and metal boning.
Rocher, London
V&A: T.53-1960

1908–10 Bust bodice. Lilac ruched silk satin.
Maker unknown, British
V&A: T.52-1960

1908–10 Bust bodice. Cream ruched silk satin.
Maker unknown, British
GALLERY OF COSTUME, MANCHESTER: 1963.315

1908–10 Feather boa. Dyed purple ostrich feather.
Maker unknown, British
V&A: T.62-1960

1908–10 Hat. Pale pink silk, trimmed with grey velvet ribbon and pale blue bird wings.
Woolland Brothers, London
V&A: T.101-1960

1908–10 Hat (plate 53). Black plaited straw trimmed with purple cotton wisteria.
Henry, London
V&A: T.105-1960

1908–10 Hat. Black felt trimmed with purple ribbon.
Woolland Brothers, London
GALLERY OF COSTUME, MANCHESTER: 1963.320

1908–10 Headdress. Silver gilt wire and diamanté.
Maker unknown, London
V&A: T.131-1960

1908–10 Headdress (plate 50). Silver gilt wire and silk laurel leaves.
Maker unknown, London
V&A: T.132-1960

1908–10 Hair comb. Tortoiseshell and silver ribbon.
Maker unknown, London
V&A: T.133-1960

1908–10 Hat (plate 147). Pale grey silk trimmed with grey ostrich feathers.
Woolland Brothers, London
V&A: CIRC.650-1964

*c.***1909** Hat. Green suede and silk braid.
René, Brighton
V&A: T.127-1960

*c.***1909** Hat. Purple suede and purple net.
Maker unknown, British
V&A: T.128-1960

*c.***1909** Tailored jacket and skirt (plate 34 – label only). Black velvet with striped silk lining.
Redfern, London
V&A: T.42&A-1960

*c.***1909** Summer afternoon dress. Cream silk and silk chiffon trimmed with machine lace and black velvet waistband.
Kate Reily, London
V&A: T.44-1960

*c.***1909** Ball dress (plates 22, 49, 126). Cream silk satin trimmed with beaded net, silver gilt lace and bugle beads.
Maker unknown, London
V&A: T.47-1960

*c.***1909** Dinner dress (plate 47). Black silk velvet with chemical-lace collar and diamanté trimmings.
Redfern, London
V&A: T.29-1960

*c.***1909** Afternoon dress (plates 46, 125). Lilac silk satin and silk chiffon trimmed with machine embroidered net.
Pickett, London
V&A: T.33-1960

*c.***1909** Blouse. White cotton.
Maker unknown, British
V&A: T.55-1960

1909–10 Summer day dress. Grey lilac linen and machine embroidery.
Maker unknown, British
V&A: T.23&A-1960

*c.***1910** Hat (plate 54). Purple silk plush trimmed with dyed fur and feathers.
Woolland Brothers
V&A: T.106-1960

*c.***1910** Hat. Black velvet with fur trim.
Woolland Brothers, London
V&A: T.107-1960

*c.***1910** Hat (plate 71). Red wool tweed motoring cap.
Woodrow, London
V&A: T.130-1960

c.1910 Evening mourning dress (plate 75). Black silk chiffon with black glass bugle beads.
Lucile, London
V&A: T.45–1960

c.1910 Handbag, powder puff and mirror (plate 120). Brown suede.
Maker unknown, London
V&A: T.72A–C–1960

c.1910 Handbag and vanity mirror. Black suede.
Maker unknown, British
V&A: CIRC.661&A–1960

c.1910 Handbag. Green suede.
Maker unknown, British
V&A: CIRC.662–1960

c.1910 Hat (plate 55). Black satin trimmed with peach satin ribbon and bird wing.
Woolland Brothers, London
V&A: T.104–1960

c.1910 Hat (plate 61 – detail). Black net trimmed with pink and black silk roses.
Woolland Brothers, London
V&A: T.114–1960

c.1910 Tailored jacket and skirt (plate 148). Navy-blue wool serge trimmed with striped blanket wool.
Woolland Brothers, London
V&A: T.37&A–1960

c.1910 Blouse (plate 41). White linen with tan trim.
Irish Linen Stores, London
V&A: T.58–1960

c.1910 Scarf. Striped mauve and black silk trimmed with silk tassels.
Maker unknown, British
V&A: T.63–1960

c.1910 Petticoat. Pleated purple silk.
Maker unknown, British
V&A: T.66–1960

c.1910 Handbag. Black suede with silk braid strap.
Maker unknown, British
V&A: T.73–1960

c.1910 Handbag. Green suede with silk tassels.
Maker unknown, British
V&A: T.74–1960

c.1910 Cape (plate 65). Dark green, brown and grey tweed with orange and blue stripe.
Scott Adie, London
V&A: T.97–1960

c.1910 Umbrella. Mauve silk with carved parrot head handle.
Maker unknown, British
V&A: T.99–1960

c.1910 Parasol. Silk and wood.
Maker unknown, British
V&A: T.100–1960

c.1910 Hat (plate 59). Black silk with pink silk flowers and ribbon.
Woolland Brothers, London
V&A: T.108–1960

c.1910 Hat (plate 60). Grey plaited straw and silk ribbon.
Woolland Brothers, London
V&A: T.120–1960

c.1910 Hat (plate 62). Black straw trimmed with ostrich feathers and dried barley.
Suzanne Talbot, Paris, for Woolland Brothers, London
V&A: T.235–1960

1910–14

1910–11 Hat. Grey felt trimmed with glacé silk.
Woolland Brothers, London
V&A: T.111–1960

1910–11 Hat. Black plaited straw trimmed with velvet and black feather.
Woolland Brothers, London
V&A: T.102–1960

1910–12 Hat. Brown leather.
René, London & Brighton
GALLERY OF COSTUME, MANCHESTER: 1963.321

1910–14 Day dress. Black serge lined with black silk.
Maker unknown, British
GALLERY OF COSTUME, MANCHESTER: 1963.301

1910–15 Nightdress. White cotton trimmed with white openwork and pink ribbon.
Maker unknown, British
GALLERY OF COSTUME, MANCHESTER: 1963.311

1910–15 Nightdress. White cotton and machine embroidery.
Maker unknown, British
GALLERY OF COSTUME, MANCHESTER: 1963.312

1910–15 Drawers. Black silk satin.
Maker unknown, British
GALLERY OF COSTUME, MANCHESTER: 1963.314

1910–15 Ice skating boots. Black leather with metal skates.
Underwood and Farrant, London
GALLERY OF COSTUME, MANCHESTER: 1963.326

1911 Tailored jacket and skirt (plate 88). Grey wool and mohair with striped silk velvet trimming.
Lucile, London
V&A: T.36&A–1960

c.1911 Hat. Black velvet trimmed with black feathers.
Michée Zac, London
V&A: T.116–1960

c.1911 Tailored jacket and skirt (plate 37). Grey woollen tweed.
Redfern, London
V&A: T.28&A–1960

c.1911 Tailored jacket and skirt (plates 35, 156). Black serge trimmed with black velvet and black jacquard woven silk braid.
Redfern, London
V&A: CIRC.647&A–1964

c.1911 Hat. Purple velour and black ribbon.
Woolland Brothers, London
V&A: CIRC.651–1964

c.1911 Hat. Black velvet trimmed with white egret feathers.
Woolland Brothers, London
V&A: CIRC.652–1964

c.1911 Tailored jacket and skirt. Grey woollen flannel with black silk velvet facings.
Redfern, London
V&A: T.39&A–1960

c.1911 'Blériot' hat (plate 56). Black straw, velvet and blue feathers.
René, Brighton
V&A: T.115–1960

c.1911 Hat. Black straw trimmed with black net and red silk rose.
Maker unknown, British
V&A: T.125–1960

1911–12 Day dress (plate 30). Lilac silk chiffon over silk trimmed with machine whitework embroidery and lace and purple silk cord.
Mascotte, London
V&A: CIRC.643–1964

1911–12 Day dress (plate 29). Mauve wool serge trimmed with ribbon and machine lace collar.
Mascotte, London
GALLERY OF COSTUME, MANCHESTER: 1963.302

1911–15 Hat. Black straw trimmed with black raffia and black silk braid.
Kate Reily, London
MUSEUM OF LONDON: 74.37/11

1912 Evening dress (plate 83). Purple silk, silk chiffon and silk satin, trimmed with metal thread and sequins, with silk tassel.
Lucile, London
V&A: T.35–1960

1912 Tailored jacket and skirt (plate 89). Grey worsted wool with silk lining.
Lucile, London
V&A: T.38&A–1960

c.1912 Summer day dress (plate 130). Mauve and white striped cotton trimmed with machine embroidered collar.
Mascotte, London
V&A: T.24–1960

c.1912 Tea coat (plate 43). Pink silk satin trimmed with net embroidered with metallic thread.
probably Lucile, London
V&A: T.48–1960

c.1912 Hat. Black velvet with black ostrich feather.
H. Taget, Paris
V&A: T.110–1960

c.1912 Dinner dress (plate 85). Black wool crêpe with black machine lace insert and cream silk banding.
Lucile, London
V&A: CIRC.645–1964

c.1912 Tea coat (plate 133). Black silk satin with silk frogging fastening and lilac satin lining.
Mascotte, London
V&A: T.98–1960

c.1912 Hat. Purple suede with purple silk braid.
René, London & Brighton
V&A: CIRC.653–1964

c.1912 Hat. Purple velvet trimmed with purple dyed ostrich feathers.
Michée Zac, London
V&A: T.118–1960

c.1912 Hat. White net and black velvet.
Woolland Brothers, London
V&A: T.119–1960

c.1912 Tailored jacket and skirt (plate 129). Purple wool serge trimmed with black silk jacquard braid.
Mascotte, London
V&A: T.43&A–1960

c.1912 Blouse (plate 42). Black silk chiffon trimmed with machine lace and silk flowers, interior chemise of silk and machine lace.
Lucile, London
V&A: T.60–1960

c.1912 Blouse (plate 39). Mauve silk chiffon trimmed with silk fringe.
Mascotte, London
V&A: T.56–1960

c.1912 Blouse. Navy silk chiffon and silk tassel trim.
Mascotte, London
MUSEUM OF LONDON: 74.37/10

1912–14 Hat. Brown silk plush and ostrich feathers.
Michée Zac, London
V&A: CIRC.655–1964

1912–14 Hat. Black velvet.
Jay's, London
V&A: CIRC.656–1964

1912–15 Nightdress. Pale pink lawn with embroidered 'Heather' motif.
Maker unknown, British
V&A: T.69–1960

1913 Evening dress (plate 87). Cream silk satin, black silk velvet and machine lace.
Lucile, London
V&A: T.31–1960

*c.*1913 Afternoon dress (plate 36). Black cashmere trimmed with purple silk crêpe.
Redfern, London
V&A: T.32–1960

*c.*1913 Afternoon dress (plates 6, 84). Ivory silk satin, silk chiffon and machine lace, trimmed with skunk fur.
Lucile, London
V&A: T.34–1960

*c.*1913 Coat (plate 117). Black double-faced blanket wool with purple cuffs, collar and buttons.
Russell & Allen, London
V&A: T.25–1960

*c.*1913 Hat (plate 58). Black straw and black waxed ribbon trimmed with white ostrich and pale pink egret feather.
Woolland Brothers, London
V&A: T.109–1960

1913–14 Tailored jacket and skirt. Herringbone tweed lined with purple satin.
Lucile, London
MUSEUM OF LONDON: 74.37/8A&B

1913–15 Hat. Black velvet and cream ribbon.
Michée Zac, London
V&A: T.121–1960

1914–20

*c.*1914 Blouse. White linen with blue trim and blue machine embroidery.
Irish Linen Stores, London
V&A: T.57–1960

*c.*1914 Blouse. Green and white striped cotton.
J.H. Gosling & Sons Ltd, London
GALLERY OF COSTUME, MANCHESTER: 1963.305

*c.*1914 'Tango' corset (plate 102). Cotton, silk satin and machine lace.
Debenham & Freebody, London
V&A: T.64–1966

1914–15 Hat. Black silk plush and black feathers.
Woolland Brothers, London
GALLERY OF COSTUME, MANCHESTER: 1963.322

1914–20 Pair of garters. Black silk satin with red silk roses.
Lucile, London
V&A: T.61–1960

*c.*1915 Cape. Black double-faced blanket wool with black and yellow lining.
Russell & Allen, London
V&A: T.16–1960

*c.*1915 Day dress. Blue linen with silk organza collar and cuffs and silk ribbon.
Maker unknown, British
V&A: T.17–1960

*c.*1915 Tailored jacket and skirt (plates 96, 99). Dark grey wool serge.
Lucile, London.
V&A: T.27&A–1960

*c.*1915 Tailored dress and jacket (plates 104, 105). Blue serge and black silk satin.
Lucile, London
V&A: T.50&A–1960

*c.*1915 Tea coat. Grey silk satin with printed silk lining.
Russell & Allen, London
V&A: CIRC.644–1964

*c.*1915 Tea coat (plates 118, 119). Lilac silk satin with printed silk lining.
Russell & Allen, London
V&A: T.46–1960

*c.*1915 Blouse. White silk with blue stripe.
Maker unknown, British
V&A: T.54–1960

*c.*1915 Tea coat. Purple ribbed silk.
Russell & Allen, London
MUSEUM OF LONDON: 74.37/5

*c.*1915 Hat. Black straw.
Woolland Brothers, London
V&A: T.126–1960

1915–18 Petticoat. Cream silk crêpe.
Maker unknown, British
GALLERY OF COSTUME, MANCHESTER: 1963.308

1915–19 Drawers. Purple and black striped silk satin.
Mrs Fane Ltd, London
V&A: T.65–1960

1915–20 Coat. Brown blanket wool.
Bradleys, London
V&A: T.18–1960

1915–20 Cardigan. Knitted silk.
Harrods, London
V&A: T.51–1960

*c.*1917 Tailored jacket and skirt (plate 98). Pale brown silk and wool.
Lucile, London
V&A: T.41&A–1960

*c.*1917 Dress. Black silk velvet trimmed with skunk fur.
Lucile, London
V&A: T.49–1960

*c.*1917 Hat. Black velvet with feather trim.
Maker unknown, British
V&A: CIRC.654–1964

*c.*1918 Skiing trousers. Navy serge with removable cotton lining.
Maker unknown, British
GALLERY OF COSTUME, MANCHESTER: 1963.306

*c.*1918 Skiing trousers. Navy wool lined with flannel.
Maker unknown, British
GALLERY OF COSTUME, MANCHESTER: 1963.308

*c.*1919 Hat. Blue silk with pink silk ribbon.
Woolland Brothers, London
V&A: T.129–1960

*c.*1919 Hat. Black silk trimmed with jacquard woven ribbon.
Maker unknown, British
V&A: CIRC.657–1964

*c.*1920 Nightdress. Pink silk and machine lace trimming.
Maker unknown, British
V&A: T.70–1960

*c.*1920 Belt. Red suede.
Maker unknown, British
V&A: T.64–1960

*c.*1920 Hat (plate 57). Straw trimmed with velvet flowers.
Lucile, London
V&A: T.113–1960

*c.*1920 Hat. Black felt plush.
Woolland Brothers, London
V&A: T.123–1960

*c.*1920 Hat. Orange felt.
Maker unknown, British
V&A: T.124–1960

1920–25

1920–25 Summer day dress (plate 103). Pink and blue striped silk.
Maker unknown, British
V&A: T.19–1960

*c.*1921 Hat. Black felt.
Woolland Bothers, London
V&A: T.112–1960

*c.*1921 Tailored jacket and skirt. Beige wool serge.
Maker unknown, British
V&A: T.40&A–1960

*c.*1925 Hat. Blue silk chiffon and gold lamé.
Woolland Brothers, London
V&A: T.122–1960

STOCKINGS

Silk, wool and cotton (some in plate 25).
V&A: T.85&A–1960 TO T.96&A–1960,
T.135&A–1960 TO T.136&A–1960 AND
CIRC.664&A–1964 TO CIRC.665&A–1964
GALLERY OF COSTUME, MANCHESTER:
1963.316&317

SHOES

Leather and suede (some in plates 149–55).
Alan McAfee, London
V&A: T.30&A–1960, T.137&A–1960,
T.138–1960, T.140&A–1960, T.147&–
1960, T.149–1960, CIRC.658&A–1964,
CIRC.659&A–1964, CIRC.660&A–1964
NORTHAMPTON MUSEUM: 1974.43.81
Leather and suede (some in plates 149–55).
Hook Knowles & Co., London
V&A: T.139&A–1960, T.141–1960,
T.142&A–1960, T.143–1960, T.144&A–1960,
T.148–1960, T.150&A–1960
NORTHAMPTON MUSEUM: 1974.43.78,
1974.43.79, 1974.43.80
GOLD LEATHER
Charles Lee, London (plate 51)
V&A: T.146&A–1960

GLOVES

Suede and kid leather (some in plate 146).
Frederick Penberthy, London
V&A: T.81&A–1960
GALLERY OF COSTUME, MANCHESTER:
1963.318
Debenham & Freebody, London
V&A: T.78&A–1960
Augustus Bide, London
V&A: T.79&A–1960, V&A: T.76&A–1960,
V&A: T.82&A–1960, V&A: T.83&A–1960, V&A:
T.84&A–1960
Made in France
V&A: CIRC.663&A–1964, V&A: T.75&A–1960,
V&A: T.77&A–1960

NOTES

Prices

All prices and values are expressed in their original pre-decimalized currency, in pounds, shillings and pence or £, s and d, in which £1 = 20s, 1s = 12d and 1 guinea = £1 1s.

Introduction

1. Madeleine Ginsburg, telephone interview, 4 March 2011. Madeleine Ginsburg acknowledges the significant contribution made to the exhibition *A Lady of Fashion* by Peter Thornton, assistant keeper, Department of Textiles, 1954–62.
2. The museum numbers for the Museum of London Firbank acquisitions are 74.37/5, 74.37/6, 74.37/7, 74.37/8a & b, 74.37/9, 74.37/10 and 74.37/11. The museum numbers for the Firbank shoes acquired by Northampton Museum are 1974.43.78, 1974.43.79, 1974.43.80 and 1974.43.81. The museum numbers for the Firbank items acquired by Nottingham Museum are NCM1974-37, NCM1974-38, NCM1974-39 and NCM1974-40.
3. Sale catalogue, 'Costume: March 19 1974. Christie's, London' (London, 1974), p.40. A selection of Heather's hats was sold to Hollywood actress Britt Ekland. Lot 247, 'A sketch book of dress designs, by Miss Firbank, pencil dated "January and February 1913"', acquired by 'Nicholson', is perhaps the most frustrating loss in terms of piecing together Heather's relationship with her clothes.
4. *A Lady of Fashion: Heather Firbank, Exh 30 Sept–4 Dec 1960*, V&A Archive file (VX.1960.006 RP/1960/1046, MA/28/106, V&A Archives).

1 · A Splendid Crescendo of Luxury

1. X. Marcel Boulestin, *Ease and Endurance, being a translation of X. Marcel Boulestin's 'A Londres naguère'* (Home and van Thal, London, 1948), p.19. Before he opened his famous restaurant, Boulestin, the most avant-garde French interior designer in London, sold products from Paul Poiret's École Martine in his Mayfair interior design studio.
2. Clare Rose, *Children's Clothes Since 1750* (B.T. Batsford, London, 1989), pp.123–7.
3. Sonia Keppel, *Edwardian Daughter* (Hamish Hamilton, London, 1958), p.41.
4. Harriette Firbank, letter to Ronald Firbank about arrangements for the day of Edward VII's Coronation, 25 May 1902, MS (Berg Collection, New York Public Library, New York).
5. Lady Firbank, letter to Ronald Firbank, December 1902, MS (Berg Collection, New York Public Library, New York).
6. Ralph Nevill (ed.), *The Reminiscences of Lady Dorothy Nevill* (Edward Arnold, London, 1906), pp.104–5.
7. Paul Thompson, *The Edwardians: The Remaking of British Society* (Routledge, London, 1992), p.4.

8. Letter from Heather Firbank to Ronald Firbank, 1903–4, written from the Coopers.
9. Catalogues and photographs relating to the sale, 'Fine Porcelain, Old French Furniture and English Furniture of Sir J. Thomas Firbank', 4–5 May 1904, V&A: Heather Firbank archive. Miriam Benkovitz records that the sale raised under '£9000': see Miriam J. Benkovitz, *Ronald Firbank: A Biography* (Weidenfeld & Nicolson, London, 1970), p.11.
10. Ronald Firbank, *The New Rhythm and Other Pieces* (Gerald Duckworth & Co., London, 1962), p.56.
11. Museum of London: Dress 74.37/6.
12. M. Dinorbin Griffith, 'At the Queen's Drawing Rooms – What Really Happens There', *Harmsworth Magazine* (February–July 1900), Vol.IV, p.357.
13. Cynthia Asquith, *Remember and Be Glad* (James Barrie, London, 1952), p.59.
14. For further information on the etiquette of court presentation see for example Mrs C.E. Humphry, *Etiquette for Every Day* (1909), available online at https://archive.org/details/cihm_66256.
15. *The Onlooker*, 23 May 1908, p.170.
16. Vita Sackville-West, *The Edwardians* (Chatto & Windus, London, 1930), p.109.
17. Cecil Beaton, *The Glass of Fashion* (Shenval Press, London, 1954), p.80.
18. Ronald Firbank, 'A Study in Temperament', in *The New Rhythm and Other Pieces* (cited in note 10), p.21.
19. Ronald Firbank, 'A Disciple from the Country' (*c.*1904), ibid., p.120.
20. Mrs Humphry, *Manners for Women* (James Bowden, London, 1897; from reprint Pryor Publication, Whitstable, 1995), p.18.

2 · The Social Whirl: A Society Wardrobe for the Season

1. Information from 1901 census: see http://ancestry.co.uk.
2. Gordon Meggy, 'The Secret of Smart Dressing', *Strand* (December 1913), p.684.
3. Lady Duff-Gordon ('Lucile'), *Discretions and Indiscretions* (Jarrolds, London, 1932), p.80.
4. Desmond Chapman-Huston (ed.), *The Private Diaries of Daisy, Princess of Pless, 1873–1914* (John Murray, London, 1950), p.114.
5. Margot Asquith, *The Autobiography of Margot Asquith* (Methuen, London, 1962), p.49.
6. Susan North, 'John Redfern and Sons, 1847–1892', *Costume: The Journal of the Costume Society*, Vol.42 (2008), pp.145–68, and 'Redfern Limited, 1892 to 1940', *Costume: The Journal of the Costume Society*, Vol.43 (2009), pp.85–108.
7. Heather's white flannel coat was sold at Christie's on 19 March 1974, Lot 206.
8. V&A: T.34–1940. This was probably made for an exhibition. A day dress by Frederick Bosworth

(*c.*1905) also survives in the collections of Leeds City Museums and Art Gallery, museum number LEEAG2012.290.7.
9. V&A: T.39&A–1960.
10. Chemical lace is a form of machine embroidery in which the supporting fabric is removed by an acid to reveal a structure of lace.
11. *Lady's Realm* (1901), p.77, quoted in Natalie Rothstein (ed.), *Four Hundred Years of Fashion* (V&A, London, 1984), p.78.
12. Vita Sackville-West, *The Edwardians* (Chatto & Windus, London, 1930), pp.34–5.
13. Cecil Beaton, *The Glass of Fashion* (Shenval Press, London, 1954), pp.13–14.
14. X. Marcel Boulestin, *Ease and Endurance, being a translation of X. Marcel Boulestin's 'A Londres naguère'* (Home and van Thal, London, 1948), p.29.
15. Ibid., p.48.
16. Cynthia Asquith, *Remember and Be Glad* (James Barrie, London, 1952), pp.165–6.
17. Letter from Cicely Mitford to Heather Firbank, *c.*1910, V&A: Heather Firbank archive.
18. Alison Adburgham, *Shops and Shopping 1800–1914: Where and in What Manner the Well-dressed Englishwoman Bought Her Clothes* (George Allen and Unwin Ltd, London, 1964), pp.73–5.
19. Heather's sporting clothes were taken in by the Gallery of English Costume (now the Gallery of Costume) in Manchester, which then held, as it does now, one of the best collections of historic sportswear in the country. As with her other garments, Heather bought from only the very best suppliers, maintaining the strict sense of propriety and fashion-consciousness that characterize the collection as a whole.
20. *Gentlewoman* (Summer 1897), quoted by Janice Helland in 'Highland Home Industries and the Fashion for Tweed', in Patrick Geddes, *Journal of the Scottish Society for Art History: The Arts and Crafts Movement*, Vol.9 (2004).
21. Helland, p.33.
22. Lucy Johnstone, 'She and Ski: The Development of Women's Ski Outfits, 1880–1930', *Costume: The Journal of the Costume Society*, Vol.38 (2004), p.91.
23. Leonard Larkin, 'Motor-cars: Yesterday and To-day', *Strand* (1913).
24. Heather's motoring coat by Woolland Brothers is in the Museum of London's collection: 74.37/7.
25. Asquith (cited in note 16), p.77.
26. Ibid.
27. Ibid., p.75.
28. Sackville-West (cited in note 12), pp.39–41.
29. Letter from Cicely Mitford to Heather Firbank, *c.*1910, V&A: Heather Firbank archive.
30. Lou Taylor, *Mourning Dress: A Costume and Social History* (Allen and Unwin, London, 1983), p.222.
31. *Evening Standard and St James's Gazette*, 10 May 1910, V&A: Heather Firbank archive.
32. Boulestin (cited in note 14), p.14.

33. Taylor (cited in note 31), p.162.
34. The authors are grateful to Lewis Orchard for kindly providing information on fashionable black Lucile gowns, including the names of specific models.
35. Taylor (cited in note 31), p.303.
36. Ronald Firbank's letter to Heather, quoted in Miriam J. Benkovitz, *Ronald Firbank: A Biography* (Weidenfeld & Nicolson, London, 1970), p.45.
37. Taylor (cited in note 31), p.303.
38. Benkovitz (cited in note 36), p.108.

3 · Discretions, Indiscretions and Nonconformity in Society London

1. Cecil Beaton, *The Glass of Fashion* (Shenval Press, London, 1954), p.32.
2. Lady Duff-Gordon ('Lucile'), *Discretions and Indiscretions* (Jarrolds, London, 1932), p.59.
3. Blanche MacManus, *The American Woman Abroad* (Dodd, Mead, 1911), p.225, available through the Internet Archive at https://archive.org/.
4. Samantha Erin Safer, 'Designing Lucile Ltd: Couture and the Modern Interior 1900–1920s', in Fiona Fisher, Trevor Keeble, Patricia Lara-Betancourt and Brenda Martin (eds), *Performance. Fashion and the Modern Interior: From the Victorians to Today* (Berg, London, 2011), pp.100–103.
5. Elizabeth Ewing, *Fur in Dress* (B.T. Batsford, London, 1981), p.22.
6. V&A museum numbers: CIRC.645–1964, T.34–1960 and T.31–1960.
7. Gordon Meggy, 'The Secret of Smart Dressing', *Strand* (December 1913), pp.680–90. The authors are grateful to Randy Bryan Bigham for drawing their attention to this article, and for highlighting an illustration of the tailored costume V&A: T.36&A–1960 (plate 88) in Vogue (US) 15 December 1911, p.33, where it is described as a 'Smart coat and skirt costume of gray ratine. The manner in which the skirt is caught up suggests the draped riding skirt and it thus shows about eight inches of the petticoat of gray satin, striped with gray velvet.'
8. Cynthia Asquith, *Remember and Be Glad* (James Barrie, London, 1952), p.70.
9. Ibid., pp.78, 103, 79, 81.
10. Elizabeth Crawford, 'Rooms of Their Own: Victorian and Edwardian Women's Clubs: A Practical Demand', *Woman and Her Sphere*, womanandhersphere.com [accessed 4 May 2014].
11. 'Women's Clubs, Truths from Inside by a Club Woman', *Girl's Own Paper Annual*, 1911–12, p.553.
12. Letter from Colonel Mitford from Arthur's, St James's Street, SW, to Heather Firbank, 23 June 1911, V&A: Heather Firbank archive.
13. 'In Society', *Daily Express*, Wednesday 24 April 1912.
14. Letter to Heather Firbank, written in French from unknown author, V&A: Heather Firbank archive.
15. Vita Sackville-West, *The Edwardians* (Chatto & Windus, London, 1930), p.26.
16. Osbert Sitwell, *Noble Essences* (Macmillan, London, 1950), p.19.
17. Philip Womack, 'Vainglory: with Inclinations and Caprice by Ronald Firbank – review', *Observer*, Sunday 5 August 2012. The reissued books were *Vainglory* (1915), *Inclinations* (1916) and *Caprice* (1917). Available at: www.guardian.co.uk/books/2012/

aug/05/vainglory-inclinations-caprice-firbank-review [accessed 23 April 2014].
18. Ibid.
19. Patricia Juliana Smith, 'Ronald Firbank', in David Scott Kestan (ed.), *The Oxford Encyclopedia of British Literature* (Oxford University Press, Oxford, 2006), p.321.
20. Ronald Firbank, *Letters to His Mother 1920–1924*, edited by Anthony Hobson (Roxburghe Club, London, 2001), pp.128 and 41.
21. Ronald Firbank, *The Artificial Princess*, in *Five Novels by Ronald Firbank* (New Directions Publishing, New York, 1981), pp.252–3.
22. *Vainglory* refers to Lucile on p.216 and *Caprice* to Redfern on p.348.
23. Letter from Lady Firbank, 44 Sloane Street, SW1, to Heather Firbank, 13 September 1919, V&A: Heather Firbank archive.
24. Firbank (cited in note 20), p. 86.
25. Letter from Heather Firbank to Ronald Firbank, 1925, V&A: Heather Firbank archive.

4 · Wartime and After: A Retreat from Society

1. *The Queen*, 11 July 1914, p.62.
2. Letter from unknown cousin, 10 Gloucester Place, to Heather Firbank, 25 August 1918, V&A: Heather Firbank archive.
3. *The Queen*, 14 November 1914, p.62.
4. Memorandum of agreement between Arthur Annesley Ronald Firbank and Lady Jane Harriette (Garrett) Firbank for the rental of Denbigh Cottage, Richmond, Surrey, 1920 (New York Public Library Archives and Manuscripts, Ronald Firbank Collection of Papers, 1896–1952). Available at: http://archives.nypl.org/brg/19141 [accessed 4 May 2014].
5. Letter from Ronald Firbank to Heather Firbank, 14 March 1922, MS (Fales Library, New York University, New York).
6. Pat Jalland, *Women, Marriage and Politics 1860–1914* (Oxford University Press, Oxford, 1986), p.260.
7. Letter from Ronald Firbank to Heather Firbank, late April/early May 1924, MS (Fales Library, New York University, New York).
8. Letter from Ronald Firbank to Heather Firbank, 4 February 1925, MS (Fales Library, New York University, New York).
9. Letter from Heather Firbank to Ronald Firbank, 22 April 1925 (Berg Collection, New York Public Library, New York).
10. Miriam J. Benkovitz, *Ronald Firbank: A Biography* (Weidenfeld & Nicolson, London, 1970), p.272.
11. Ibid., pp.194–5.
12. Several sources, including the press release for the V&A exhibition *A Lady of Fashion*, state that Heather Firbank deposited her clothes in 1921. However, a letter in the V&A Archive files reveals that they were actually deposited in 1926. Midland Bank Chambers, letter to Madeleine Ginsburg, 6 September 1960, TS (*A Lady of Fashion: Heather Firbank, Exh 30 Sept–4 Dec 1960*, V&A Archive file (VX.1960.006 RP/1960/1046, MA/28/106, V&A Archives).
13. Letter sold in 2012 by Adam Andrusier Autographs, Pinner, London, signed by Daphne Du Maurier. With thanks to Joe Taylor.
14. *Grace's Guide to Industrial History* (Bradley's, the Arctic Fur Store). Available at:

http://www.gracesguide.co.uk/Bradleys%27 (The Arctic Fur Store).
15. On 2 August 1938, she paid Daimler Hire Ltd of Hove four guineas and a further £4 12s 6d was sent to Chrysler Motors on 14 April 1939. On 1 July 1937, she had been obliged to pay £9 7s 2d to a tyre company.
16. Heather Firbank's death certificate describes her as 'Spinster, of Independent Means, Daughter of Joseph Thomas Firbank, Knight, MP (retired) (deceased)'. She died of a cerebral haemorrhage at the nursing home on 13 April 1954. Her funeral was organized by Hiltons, a local undertakers, following instructions from Martin James Pollock, solicitors, of Howard Street, the Strand. With thanks to Richard Bryant, Lindfield Historical Society, and Joanna Friel, Chislehurst Historical Society.

5 · Heather Firbank and London's Couture Industry

1. 'She has dressed 3 Coronations and 32 Courts – Mrs Mortimer of Worth', *Housewife* (June 1953). Available at: sheepandchick.blogspot.co.uk/2012/07/mrs-mortimer-of-worth.html [accessed 14 July 2012].
2. 'Houses of Fashion', *Observer*, 30 October 1910.
3. 'Soon I was in virtual paroxysms of impatience while awaiting my father to bring home the paper in which this lady's latest pen drawing would be ready to be smeared with my water-colours or oddly smelling silver and gold paints', Cecil Beaton, *The Glass of Fashion* (Shenval Press, London, 1954), p.15.
4. See the article 'Beware the cape and the exaggeratedly long tunic, unless you are tall and slender', *New York Tribune*, Sunday 31 May 1914.
5. Erika Diane Rappaport, *Shopping for Pleasure: Women in the Making of London's West End* (Princeton University Press, Princeton, NJ, 2000), p.9.
6. Virginia Woolf, *Mrs Dalloway* (Grafton Books, London, 1978), p.12.
7. The Lafayette Archive, V&A Photographic Studio. Available at: http://lafayette.org.uk/gee2059.html [accessed 26 August 2014]. A group of garments by Russell & Allen also survives in the collection at Glasgow Museums: E.1978.52.2, E.1988.104.4 and E.1988.104.5.
8. Cynthia Asquith, *Remember and Be Glad* (James Barrie, London, 1952), pp.75–6. Asquith's favourite milliner Louise Piers is likely to be Louise de Kerrighan Piers, who appears in the 1911 census as a milliner at 6 Halkin Street, Grosvenor Place. There is no currently known evidence that this milliner was connected with the large firm of Louise & Co. and Maison Lewis of Regent Street, where Heather was a customer. Asquith's favourite dressmaker, Madame Marie Marte, is listed in Post Office directories at 58 Conduit Street.
9. Lady Angela Forbes, *Memories and Base Details* (Hutchinson, London, 1921), pp.58–9. Available at: http://archive.org/stream/memoriesbasedeta00forbuoft/.
10. Letter from Worth (London), 29 November 1910, private collection. This highlights the expense of French couture compared to Heather Firbank's most expensive dress according to her bills, a 'Black velvet mousseline Gown', which she bought from Redfern for £27 6s on 20 November 1909 (see pl.112).
11. Some details about the workings of this firm are provided by the reminiscences of Marguerite Shoobert, a model who worked for Kate Reily and

other court dressmakers from 1906. See Lou Taylor, 'Marguerite Shoobert, London Fashion Model, 1906–1917', *Costume: The Journal of the Costume Society*, Vol.17 (1983), pp.105–10.

12. Gallery of Costume, Manchester (1947.3965), National Museums of Northern Ireland (BELUM. T2157: Ulster Museum), Fine Art Museum San Francisco (785644a–b) and Staten Island Historical Society (CO1.3304). The V&A collection also includes a fashion doll dressed in an afternoon dress of c.1903 (V&A: T.23–1943).

13. The marriage of Lord William Nevill and Miss Luisa Carmen de Murrieta at Brompton Oratory on 12 February 1889 was reported in the *New York Times* on 7 April 1889.

14. Taylor (cited in note 11).

15. The entry for Major Arthur George Frederick Griffiths in the *Oxford Dictionary of National Biography* refers to his marriage to Harriet, daughter of Richard Reily, but makes no mention of his wife's equally fascinating career.

16. *Pall Mall Gazette*, 26 May 1909, quoted in Rappaport (cited in note 5), p.131.

17. *Leeds Mercury*, 9 May 1881, and *Morning Post*, 4 July 1899.

18. *London American Register*, 22 November 1884.

19. *Hampshire Telegraph and Sussex Chronicle*, 15 October 1887.

20. *New York Times*, 1 November 1894.

21. *New York Times*, 5 March 1892.

22. Lady Duff-Gordon ('Lucile'), *Discretions and Indiscretions* (Jarrolds, London, 1932), p.67, and 'Reminiscences of a Court Dressmaker: Miss Emily Phillips interviewed by Janet Arnold in January 1974', *Costume: The Journal of the Costume Society*, 8 (1974), pp.22–5.

23. For example, *Country Life*, 27 October 1900.

24. 'Seen at the Shops', *Observer*, 25 April 1909.

25. For instance, Mrs Dunstan of New York. Family historian Graham Lines has discovered that the maker of spectacular dresses in the collections of the Metropolitan Museum, New York, and the Philadelphia Museum of Art was in fact Alice Mary Burton (1862–1927), a dressmaker from London, whose husband, James Webber Dunstan, was a dressmaker's clerk, according to the 1881 census, at 100 Mount Street, an address previously occupied by Kate Reily. Graham Lines's research shows that between 1890 and 1913 Mr and Mrs Dunstan travelled from Southampton to New York each spring and autumn. Mr Dunstan's trade was 'Dress Goods Importer', and his wife became very well known, as is shown by her highest-profile commission: providing in 1906 the wedding dress of Miss Alice Roosevelt, President Theodore Roosevelt's daughter.

26. *Grantham Journal*, 16 August 1890. Museum of London object numbers 33.174 and 36.1X1.

27. It has not been possible as yet to trace Sarah Rossiter in the census records.

28. See note 1. Business details taken from Anne Kjellberg and Susan North, *Style & Splendour: The Wardrobe of Queen Maud of Norway 1896–1938* (V&A, London, 2005), p.58 and notes.

29. Letter from the Hon. Sybelle Crossley to Madeleine Ginsburg, 5 August 1960, *A Lady of Fashion: Heather Firbank, Exh 30 Sept–4 Dec 1960*, V&A Archive file (VX.1960.006 RP/1960/1046, MA/28/106, V&A Archives).

30. Amy de la Haye, Eleanor Thompson and Lou Taylor, *A Family of Fashion: The Messels:*

Six Generations of Dress (Philip Wilson Publishers, London, 2005), p.79.

31. 'For and About Women', *Evening Standard and St James's Gazette*, 25 March 1914, V&A: Heather Firbank archive.

32. See sale catalogue for other examples of Heather's purchases from Mascotte, current whereabouts unknown: 'Costume: March 19 1974. Christie's, London' (London, 1974).

33. 'Barkers will sell the stock of Maison Mascotte', *Daily Mail*, Saturday 23 February 1918.

34. Ibid.

35. 'Madame Machinka has returned to 8 Conduit Street from Paris with her New Models', *Morning Post*, Monday 17 January 1897. The collection at Brighton Museum and Art Gallery includes an evening dress by Machinka owned by Lady Desborough (CT004807).

36. 'The Nobility and Trade', *Aberdeen Journal*, Monday 24 June 1907. Other dressmakers mentioned under the same heading are Vanité, Madame Rita, Madame de Courcy, Maison Lucille and Vera.

37. See note 2.

38. 'I was almost born on the steps of a Court Dressmaker', Hardy Amies, *Just So Far* (Collins, London, 1954), p.17.

39. E.P. Thompson and Eileen Yeo (eds), *The Unknown Mayhew: Selection from the Morning Chronicle 1849–1850* (Merlin Press, London, 1971) and Henry Mayhew, *London Labour and the London Poor*, ed. Victor Neuburg (Penguin, Harmondsworth, 1985).

40. Mrs C.S. Peel, *The Hat Shop* (John Lane, Bodley Head, London, 1914), pp.15–16.

41. Ibid.

42. 'Interview with managers of Dressmaking and Millinery depts., Messrs Jones Bros, Holloway Road, N.', 'Charles Booth and the survey into life and labour in London (1886–1903)', B112 1 056, London School of Economics & Political Science.

43. On 28 March 1913, under the headline 'A Milliner's Salary', the *Evening Post* reported on a court case brought by Miss Reska Fromatt Ospovat against her former employers, Messrs Wilson of Hanover Square, who had dismissed her after she injured a finger during a flying accident. Miss Ospovat earned the considerable sum of £800 a year. Available at: paperspast.natlib.govt.nz [accessed 28 February 2014].

44. See, for example, on the reverse of design for V&A: T.35–1960 (see pl.82), V&A: Archive of Art and Design, AAD/2008/6/22.

45. Asquith (cited in note 8), p.55.

46. Letter from Mrs S.B. Jarrett to Madeleine Ginsburg, 10 August 1960: 'I remember the name of Miss Heather Firbank but cannot recall her features … I am sorry I have no souvenirs but I have my wedding dress and veil which were made in madam's workrooms – copied from a model. I could lend you these.' *A Lady of Fashion: Heather Firbank, Exh 30 Sept–4 Dec 1960*, V&A Archive file (VX.1960.006 RP/1960/1046, MA/28/106).

47. Asquith (cited in note 8), p.75.

48. Woolland Brothers bill, July 1909 and 15 October 1910, V&A: Heather Firbank archive.

49. From 'Knightsbridge South Side: East of Sloane Street: William Street to Sloane Street', *Survey of London*, Vol.45: Knightsbridge (English Heritage, London, 2000), pp.29–36. Available at: http://www.british-history.ac.uk/report [accessed 20 December 2012].

50. The bill lists two cardigans and 11 felt hats, which added about £20 to her running account of over £400.

51. Woodrow & Sons bill, 25 September 1909, V&A: Heather Firbank archive.

52. 'High Art in Dress. London and Paris in Competition at Earl's Court', *Observer*, 26 January 1908.

53. 'Seen at the Shops', *Observer*, 26 January 1908.

54. *Ladies Field*, 7 December 1907.

55. Kenneth Florey, *Women's Suffrage Memorabilia: An Illustrated Historical Study* (Jefferson, North Carolina, 2013), p.106.

56. 'Summer Sales: Where to Secure Bargains – by Mrs Jack May', *Observer*, 27 June 1915.

57. Asquith (cited in note 8), p.75.

58. Jenny Morris, *Women Workers in the Sweated Trades: The Origins of Minimum Wage Legislation* (Gower, Aldershot, 1986).

59. See note 42.

60. Christina Walkley, *The Ghost in the Looking Glass: The Victorian Seamstress* (Peter Owen, London, 1981), 'Charles Booth and the survey into life and labour in London (1886–1903)', B112 1 056, London School of Economics & Political Science, and Mary Neal 'Dressmaking' in the 'Sweated Industries Exhibition', 1906, exh. cat. Museum of London archives.

61. 'For and About Women', *Evening Standard and St James's Gazette*, 11 July 1910, V&A: Heather Firbank archive.

62. See Joel H. Kaplan and Sheila Stowell, *Theatre and Fashion: Oscar Wilde to the Suffragettes* (Cambridge University Press, Cambridge, 1994), and Michele Majer (ed.), *Staging Fashion, 1880–1920* (Bard Graduate Center, New York, 2012). Christopher Breward, '"At home" at the St James's: Dress, Décor and the Problem of Fashion in Edwardian Theatre', in Fiona Fisher, Trevor Keeble, Patricia Lara-Betancourt and Brenda Martin (eds), *Performance, Fashion and the Modern Interior* (Berg Publishers, London, 2011), pp.83–96.

63. Norman Hartnell, *Silver and Gold* (Evans Brothers, London, 1955), p.17.

64. Mrs. C.S. Peel, *Life's Enchanted Cup* (John Lane, London, 1933), p.117.

Conclusion

1. Lady Duff-Gordon ('Lucile'), *Discretions and Indiscretions* (Jarrolds, London, 1932), p.42.

2. George G. Iggers, *Historiography in the Twentieth Century: From Scientific Objectivity to the Postmodern Challenge* (Wesleyan University Press, Hanover, 2005), p.103.

3. Gaynor Kavanagh (ed.), *Making Histories in Museums* (Leicester University Press, London, 1996), p.13.

4. Interview with Johanna Firbank, 24 April 2013.

5. Ibid.

FURTHER READING

Alison Adburgham, *Shops and Shopping 1800–1914: Where and in What Manner the Well-dressed Englishwoman Bought Her Clothes* (George Allen and Unwin Ltd, London, 1964)

Cynthia Asquith, *Remember and Be Glad* (James Barrie, London, 1952)

Cecil Beaton, *The Glass of Fashion* (Shenval Press, London, 1954)

Miriam J. Benkovitz, *Ronald Firbank: A Biography* (Weidenfeld & Nicolson, London, 1970)

Randy Bryan Bigham, *Lucile: Her Life by Design* (MacEvie Press Group, San Francisco, 2012)

Leonore Davidoff, *The Best Circles: Society Etiquette and the Season* (Croom Helm, London, 1973)

Amy de la Haye, Lou Taylor and Eleanor Thompson, *A Family of Fashion: The Messels. Six Generations of Dress* (Philip Wilson Publishers, London, 2005)

Lady Duff-Gordon ('Lucile'), *Discretions and Indiscretions* (Jarrolds, London 1932)

Caroline Evans, *The Mechanical Smile: Modernism and the First Fashion Shows in France and America 1900–1929* (Yale University Press, New Haven, 2013)

Elizabeth Ewing, *History of 20th Century Fashion* (Batsford, London, 1974)

Ronald Firbank, *Letters to His Mother 1920–1924*, edited by Anthony Hobson (Roxburghe Club, London, 2001)

Fiona Fisher, Trevor Keeble, Patricia Lara-Betancourt and Brenda Martin (eds), *Performance, Fashion and the Modern Interior: From the Victorians to Today*, (Berg, London, 2011)

Pat Jalland, *Women, Marriage and Politics 1860–1914* (Oxford University Press, Oxford, 1986)

Anne Kjellberg and Susan North, *Style & Splendour: The Wardrobe of Queen Maud of Norway 1896–1938* (V&A, London, 2005)

Valerie D. Mendes and Amy de la Haye, *Lucile Ltd. London, Paris, New York and Chicago 1892–1930s* (V&A, London, 2009)

Susan North, 'Redfern Limited, 1892 to 1940', *Costume: The Journal of the Costume Society*, Vol.43 (2009)

Adelheid Rasche, *Wardrobes in Wartime: Fashion and Fashion Image during the First World War, 1914–1918* (E.A. Seemann, Leipzig, 2014)

Vita Sackville-West, *The Edwardians* (Chatto & Windus, London, 1930)

Lou Taylor, *Mourning Dress: A Costume and Social History* (Allen and Unwin, London, 1983)

ARCHIVE MATERIAL

AAD Lucile archive, V&A, London

AAD Heather Firbank archive, V&A, London

Heather Firbank, *Letters to Ronald Firbank*, Ronald Firbank Collection of papers, 1896–1952, Berg Collection (MSS Firbank), New York Public Library, New York

Ronald Firbank, *Letters to Heather Firbank*, Fales Manuscript Collection *c.*1700–2000 (MSS001), Fales Library, New York University, New York

PICTURE CREDITS

Plate 5 Archive Photos/Stringer (Photo by Warner Brothers/Getty Images)

Plate 6 © National Portrait Gallery, London

Plate 29 © Manchester Art Gallery, UK

Plates 33, 121, 124, 127, 134, 143 © English Heritage

Plate 74 Topical Press Agency/Stringer (Photo by Topical Press Agency/Getty Images)

Plate 78 © John Culme's Footlights Notes Collection

Plate 86 © The British Library Board

Plate 108 Courtesy of D. Sharp

Plate 109 From the James Gray Collection, the photographic archive of the Regency Society, www.regencysociety.org

Plate 115 Science & Society Picture Library/Contributor (Photo by Science & Society Picture Library/SSPL/Getty Images)

Plates 139, 140 Given by John Culme, 1996 © National Portrait Gallery, London

ACKNOWLEDGEMENTS

This book is the result of collaboration between three authors, Cassie Davies-Strodder and Jenny Lister, curators in the Fashion and Textiles department at the V&A, and Lou Taylor, Professor of Dress and Textile History at the University of Brighton. Its origins lie in research undertaken by Cassie Davies-Strodder for her MA thesis, 'Creating Illusions: An Analysis of the Distribution, Use and Interpretation of the Heather Firbank Collection at the Victoria and Albert Museum, London (1957–2011)', at the University of Brighton. Lou Taylor provided much of the research into the complex social context for Heather's clothing and in particular into Heather's later life. Jenny Lister's investigation into the London shops and dressmakers Heather patronized is presented here for the first time. The book has been edited by Cassie Davies-Strodder and Jenny Lister.

We are also grateful to the many people who have helped with the research for and production of this publication. It would not have been possible without the support of Christopher Wilk and Claire Wilcox of the Furniture, Textiles and Fashion department, and Mark Eastment of V&A Publishing. Particular thanks are due to Edwina Ehrman, and other colleagues who have been generous with their expertise and enthusiasm are Elizabeth Bisley, Clare Browne, Oriole Cullen, Max Donnelly, Hanne Faurby, Sarah Medlam, Daniel Milford-Cottam, Lesley Miller, Susan North, Louise Rytter, Jana Scholze and Stephanie Wood.

Most of the beautiful illustrations of Heather Firbank's clothes and accessories are thanks to Rachael Lee's skilled and sensitive conservation and mounting and Jaron James's stylish photography. We also thank Richard Davis of the V&A Photographic Studio and, from the conservation department, Marion Kite, Frances Hartog, Joanne Hackett and Keira Miller. Thanks are also due to Christopher Marsden and Victoria Platt of the Archive of Art and Design, Sally Williams and colleagues of the National Art Library, Clare Phillips of the Metalwork department and Roisin Inglesby and Bronwen Colquhoun of the Paintings, Drawings and Prints department for their help.

We acknowledge the team at V&A Publishing, especially our editor, Philip Contos, and Anjali Bulley, Zara Anvari, Davina Cheung and Clare Davis. Lesley Levene was invaluable as a copy-editor, and we have enjoyed seeing the development of Robert Dalrymple's intelligent and appealing book design.

Many others have contributed to the research presented here. Beatrice Behlen, Curator of Fashion and Textiles at the Museum of London, and Kay Staniland, one of her predecessors there, Miles Lambert of the Gallery of Costume, Jane May of Leicester Museum and Andrew King of Nottingham Museum provided access to and information on Heather Firbank garments in their collections. Martin Pel of Brighton Museum, Rebecca Quinton of Glasgow Museums, Natalie Raw of Leeds City Museums and Art Galleries and Pauline Rushton of National Museums Liverpool shared details of garments made by Heather's dressmakers in these museums. Susan Mayor, former dress specialist at Christie's, provided information about the 1974 sale of Heather Firbank garments. Rachel Greer of the Fales Library, New York, and Anne Garner of the New York Public Library facilitated access to the Firbank family letters in their collections.

The chapter on Heather Firbank and the London couture industry has drawn considerably on painstaking research completed by Camilla de Winton and Keren Protheroe, and their work is gratefully acknowledged. Amy de la Haye and Sue Kerry also contributed helpful information. Randy Bryan Bigham and Lewis Orchard were extremely generous with their extraordinary knowledge of Lucile designs and John Culme kindly allowed us to use his image of 23 Hanover Square. We would also like to thank Vanessa Jones for tireless work in sorting and cataloguing the Firbank archive material.

We thank Madeleine Ginsburg as the first Curator of Dress at the V&A for acquiring the Heather Firbank Collection and archive and for her initial research into Lucile and Heather's other dressmakers, as well as her continued interest in this project. The book has been written with the support of the Firbank family and the authors would like to express particular gratitude to Johanna Firbank.

INDEX

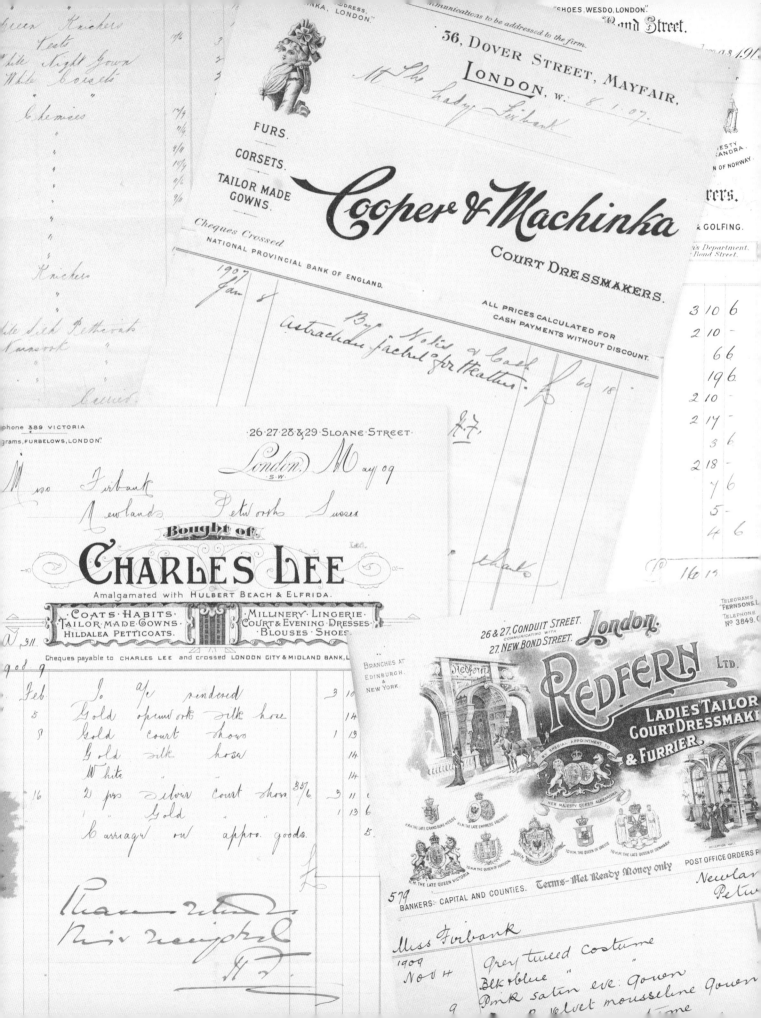

green Knickers
Vests
White Night Gown
White Corsets
"

Chemises

Knickers

White Silk Petticoats
Nainsook

Carried

"SHOES, WESDO, LONDON."
Bond Street.

Communications to be addressed to the firm.

36, DOVER STREET, MAYFAIR,
LONDON, W.

To The Lady Firbank

FURS.
CORSETS.
TAILOR MADE GOWNS.

Cheques Crossed
NATIONAL PROVINCIAL BANK OF ENGLAND.

Cooper & Machinka

COURT DRESSMAKERS.

ALL PRICES CALCULATED FOR
CASH PAYMENTS WITHOUT DISCOUNT.

1907
Jan 8

By Notis & back
Astrachan jacket for Heather £60 18

GOLFING.

's Department.
Bond Street.

3 10 6
2 10 -
6 6
19 6
2 10 -
2 17 -
3 6
2 18 -
7 6
5 -
4 6

16 15

Phone 389 VICTORIA
grams, FURBELOWS, LONDON."

26·27·28 & 29 · SLOANE · STREET

London May 09
S.W.

Miss Firbank
Newlands Petworth Sussex

Bought of
CHARLES LEE
Amalgamated with HULBERT BEACH & ELFRIDA.

COATS · HABITS.   MILLINERY · LINGERIE.
TAILOR MADE GOWNS.   COURT & EVENING DRESSES.
HILDALEA PETTICOATS.   BLOUSES · SHOES.

Cheques payable to CHARLES LEE and crossed LONDON CITY & MIDLAND BANK,

311

908 9
Feb   To a/c rendered   3 10
5   Gold open work silk hose   14
8   Gold court shoes   1 13
    Gold silk hose   14
    White "   14
16 2 prs silver court shoes 35/6 3 11
    1 " Gold   1 13 6
    Carriage on appro. goods.   5

Please return

BRANCHES AT
EDINBURGH
&
NEW YORK.

TELEGRAMS
FERNSONS, L
TELEPHONE
No 3849

26 & 27 CONDUIT STREET.   London
COMMUNICATING WITH
27. NEW BOND STREET.

REDFERN LTD

LADIES' TAILOR
COURT DRESSMAKE
& FURRIER.

BY SPECIAL APPOINTMENT TO
HER MAJESTY QUEEN ALEXANDRA

BANKERS: CAPITAL AND COUNTIES.   Terms—Net Ready Money only

POST OFFICE ORDERS P

Newlar
Petw

579

Miss Firbank
1909   Grey tweed Costume
Nov 4   Blk & blue "
         Pink satin eve gown
9   velvet mousseline gown

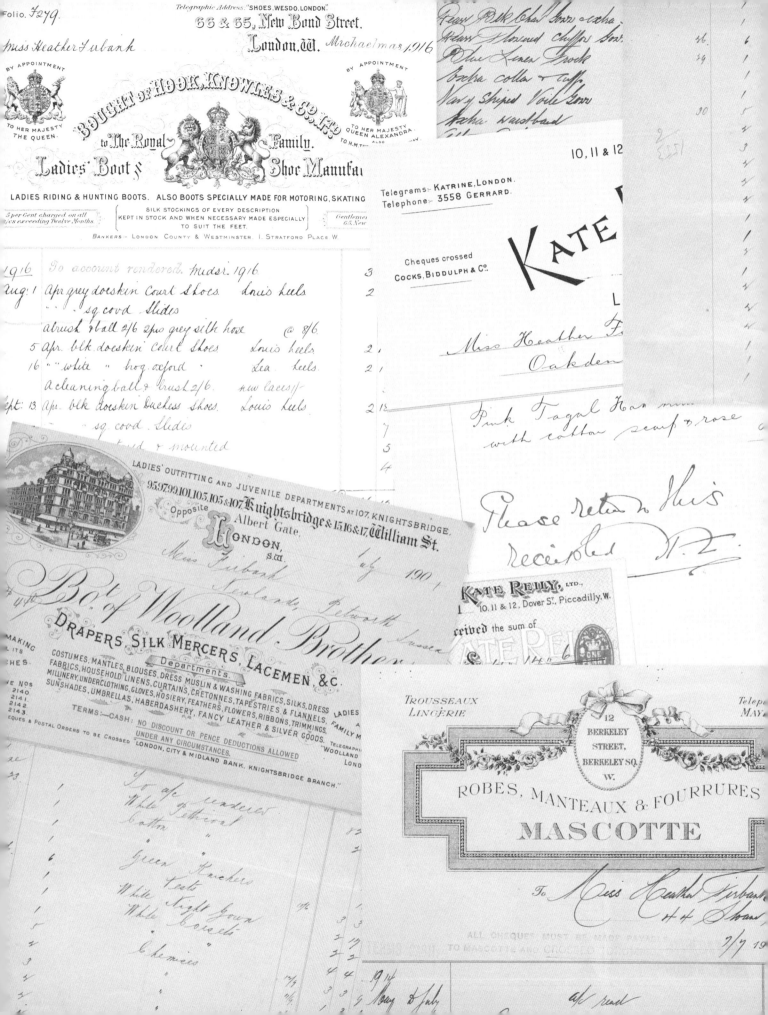

Folio. 7279.

Miss Heather Eubank

BY APPOINTMENT
TO HER MAJESTY
THE QUEEN.

BOUGHT OF HOOK, KNOWLES & CO LTD
to The Royal — Family.
Ladies' Boot & Shoe Manufa...

BY APPOINTMENT
TO HER MAJESTY
QUEEN ALEXANDRA.
ALSO
TO H.M. TH...

LADIES RIDING & HUNTING BOOTS. ALSO BOOTS SPECIALLY MADE FOR MOTORING, SKATING

5 per Cent charged on all ...cs exceeding Twelve Months.

SILK STOCKINGS OF EVERY DESCRIPTION
KEPT IN STOCK AND WHEN NECESSARY MADE ESPECIALLY
TO SUIT THE FEET.

Gentlemen
65 New

BANKERS - LONDON COUNTY & WESTMINSTER, I. STRATFORD PLACE W.

1916 To account rendered. Midsr. 1916

Aug: 1 Apr grey doeskin Court Shoes.   Louis heels
        ... sq covd Slides
        a brush & ball 2/6 2 prs grey silk hose   @ 8/6
  5 Apr. blk doeskin court shoes   Louis heels
 16 " white " hog oxford ·   Lea heels.
        a cleaning ball & brush 2/6.   new laces/
Sept: 13 Apr. blk doeskin Duchess shoes.   Louis heels
        — sq covd Slides
        ... ed & mounted

Cheques crossed
Cocks, Biddulph & Co.

KATE

Miss Heather F...
Oakden

Pink Tagal Ha...
with cotton scarf & rose

Please return this
Receipted. N.Z.

KATE REILLY LTD.,
10, 11 & 12, Dover St., Piccadilly, W.
...ceived the sum of

LADIES' OUTFITTING AND JUVENILE DEPARTMENTS at 107, KNIGHTSBRIDGE.
93, 95, 97, 99, 101, 103, 105 & 107 Knightsbridge & 15, 16 & 17, William St.
Opposite Albert Gate,
London, S.W.

Miss Eubank
Newlands, Petworth
Sussex

190...

Bot of Woolland Brothers

DRAPERS, SILK MERCERS, LACEMEN, &C.

Departments.

COSTUMES, MANTLES, BLOUSES, DRESS MUSLIN & WASHING FABRICS, SILKS, DRESS
FABRICS, HOUSEHOLD LINENS, CURTAINS, CRETONNES, TAPESTRIES, & FLANNELS.
MILLINERY, UNDERCLOTHING, GLOVES, HOSIERY, FEATHERS, FLOWERS, RIBBONS, TRIMMINGS,
SUNSHADES, UMBRELLAS, HABERDASHERY, FANCY LEATHER & SILVER GOODS.

TERMS:—CASH: NO DISCOUNT OR PENCE DEDUCTIONS ALLOWED
UNDER ANY CIRCUMSTANCES.
...eques & Postal Orders to be Crossed LONDON, CITY & MIDLAND BANK, KNIGHTSBRIDGE BRANCH."

To a/c rendered
White Petticoat
...otton
Green Knickers
...Vests
White Night Gown
White Corsets
Chemies

TROUSSEAUX
LINGERIE

12
BERKELEY
STREET,
BERKELEY SQ.
W.

ROBES, MANTEAUX & FOURRURES
MASCOTTE

To Miss Heather Eubank
44 Sloane...

ALL CHEQUES MUST BE MADE PAYABLE ...
TO MASCOTTE AND CROSSED...

1914
May & July